Critical Issues in
Gastroenterology

Critical Issues in
Gastroenterology

edited by

GARY GITNICK, MD

Department of Medicine
Division of Digestive Disorders
UCLA School of Medicine
Center for the Health Sciences
Los Angeles, California

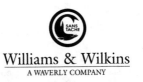

Williams & Wilkins
A WAVERLY COMPANY

BALTIMORE • PHILADELPHIA • LONDON • PARIS • BANGKOK
BUENOS AIRES • HONG KONG • MUNICH • SYDNEY • TOKYO • WROCLAW

Editor: Jonathan W. Pine, Jr.
Managing Editor: Keith Rhett Murphy
Marketing Manager: Lorraine A. Smith
Production Coordinator: Raymond E. Reter
Project Editor: Ulita Lushnycky
Designer Coordinator: Mario Fernandez
Typesetter/Digitized Illustrations: Peirce Graphic Services, Inc.
Printer/Binder: Vicks Lithograph & Printing Corp.

Printed in the United States of America

Library of Congress Cataloging-in-Publication Data

Critical issues in gastroenterology / edited by Gary Gitnick.
     p.   cm.
    Includes bibliographical references and index.
    ISBN 0–683–30555–7
      1. Gastrointestinal system—Diseases—Miscellanea.
   2. Gastroenterology—Miscellanea.   3. Colon (Anatomy)—Cancer—Miscellanea.   I. Gitnick, Gary L.
    [DNLM: 1. Colonic Diseases, Functional—therapy.   2. Hepatitis C—therapy.   3. Colonic Neoplasms—therapy.   4. Proton Pump—antagonists & inhibitors.   WI 520 C934 1998]
    RC802.C655 1998
    616.393—dc21
    DNLM/DLC   97–43319
    for Library of Congress   CIP

                                     98 99 00 01 02
                            1 2 3 4 5 6 7 8 9 10

Dedication

This book is dedicated to all those who have made my work possible—to my mother **Ann**; my wife **Cherna**; my brother **Jerry** and his wife **Saranne**; and my children and their spouses, **Neil** and **Anita**, **Kim** and **Richard**, **Jill** and **Seth**, and **Tracy** and **Stewart**.

Preface

As the editor of this book, I have enlisted authors to present an up-to-date account of issues that are of critical importance in gastroenterology. It is our hope that these chapters will be of value to primary care physicians as well as to surgeons and gastroenterologists. To develop this text, we reviewed modern literature that emphasized areas in which rapid change has occurred and is occurring. On this basis, many more specialized subjects have been excluded. Growth in basic and clinical gastroenterology remains exponential. The progress has been so great that no one author has the knowledge that covers the entire field. Although multiple authors may have led to unnecessary duplication of information, we attempted to avoid these problems by having the manuscript undergo an extensive review and rigorous editing process.

My goal for this book remains to develop a volume of manageable size, which is current and provides information on the cutting edge of gastroenterology. My hope is not only to provide state of the art information in critical areas, but also to define areas where knowledge is insufficient or where controversy is rampant. In this way, *Critical Issues in Gastroenterology* can stimulate investigators, students, and clinicians to pursue the many unsolved problems that remain in gastroenterology.

GARY GITNICK, M.D.

Acknowledgments

The authors and editor are grateful to Barbara Caganich for her dedicated efforts in organizing the manuscripts for this text. Her efficient and pleasant manner made it possible to keep this assessment of clinical issues current. We are also indebted to Keith Murphy of Williams and Wilkins for managing the development of this book and bringing it to publication.

Contributor List

Gary Gitnick, MD
Ray and Fran Stark Foundation
Professor of Medicine
Chief, Division of Digestive Diseases
UCLA School of Medicine
Los Angeles, California

Steve Fullerton, MPH
Research Specialist
Section Head, Health Services
Research
Division of Digestive Diseases
UCLA School of Medicine
Los Angeles, California

Melvyn G. Korman, MD
Director of Gastroenterology
Professor of Medicine
Monash Medical Centre
Victoria, Australia

Fiona B. Nicholson, MD
Senior Fellow, Gastroenterology
Unit
Monash Medical Centre
Victoria, Australia

Emeran A. Mayer, MD
Professor of Medicine and Physiology
Section Head, UCLA/CURE
Neuroenteric Disease Program
Division of Digestive Diseases
UCLA School of Medicine
Los Angeles, California

Lin Chang, MD
Adjunct Assistant Professor of
Medicine
UCLA School of Medicine
UCLA/CURE Neuroenteric
Disease Program
Los Angeles, California

Tony Lembo, MD
Department of Medicine
Division of Gastroenterology
Beth Israel Deaconess Medical
Center
Instructor of Medicine
Harvard Medical School
Boston, Massachussetts

Geetanjali A. Akerkar, MD
Gastroenterology Fellow
Division of Gastroenterology
Veterans Affairs Medical Center
San Francisco, California

Teresa L. Wright, MD
Associate Professor of Medicine
University of California, San
Francisco
Chief, Gastroenterology
Veterans Affairs Medical
Center
San Francisco, California

John H. Bond, MD
Professor of Medicine
University of Minnesota
Chief, Gastroenterology
Section
Minneapolis VA Medical Center
Minneapolis, Minnesota

Lee S. Rosen, MD
Clinical Instructor
Director, Cancer Therapy
Development Program
UCLA Division of Hematology-
Oncology
Los Angeles, California

Contents

Chapter One

STRATEGIC PLANNING FOR MANAGED CARE

Steve Fullerton, MPH

INTRODUCTION

The business community has long recognized strategic planning as one of the key determinants of success. In recent years, strategic planning has been acknowledged and adopted by nonprofit organizations as standard practice. Historically, medicine has been insulated from the market forces that determine financial profit and loss, but this is no longer the case in today's environment of limited resources and economic constraint. Today, managed care is rapidly replacing the traditional fee-for-service system of health care delivery.

Recent US statistics illustrate the economic impact of medical care for gastrointestinal (GI) conditions. In 1985, the direct medical care cost for patients with digestive diseases was more than 40 billion dollars, which accounted for more than 10% of all US medical care expenditures. This figure translates to approximately 1.5% of the total US gross national product. In addition to direct medical care, individuals spent a lot of money on non-medical health care for GI problems. A recent study of overall health care spending indicated Americans made an estimated 425 million visits to providers of unconventional therapy in 1990. Total medical expenditures associated with use of unconventional therapy amounted to approximately 13.7 billion dollars, approximately 75% of which was paid out-of-pocket. Due to the chronic nature of many GI conditions and the high prevalence of GI conditions, it is likely a large proportion of this non-medical health care expenditure by individuals is for digestive conditions. Indirect costs are also high. Another US survey estimated more than 158 million restricted-activity days and 22 million work-loss days are reported annually by persons with digestive diseases. The rate for work-loss days is 3 to 4 times the absenteeism rate reported by the rest of the workforce.

Strategic planning can be used to guide individuals and organizations during periods of rapid change. Strategic planning is a tool that can be used by practicing gastroenterologists to take advantage of changes in the medical care system to ensure future success. This chapter provides an overview of strategic planning concepts for gastroenterologists and explores four major areas of change in the field of gastroenterology that are occurring as a result of the rapid transition to managed care. The four areas outlined are 1) practice-based clinical trials, 2) outcomes research, 3) clinical practice guidelines, and 4) disease management.

STRATEGIC PLANNING

Today's health care marketplace is highly competitive, and the changing business and regulatory climates are making it even more difficult for gastroenterologists to compete. However, these changes are also creating new opportunities. Major areas of opportunity that are emerging include: involvement of the private practitioner in testing and evaluating new therapeutic compounds, research studies measuring the quality of care and patient outcomes, systematic improvement in the process of care, and the development and evaluation of new models of health care delivery. Gastroenterologists who are able to take advantage of these opportunities will be better equipped to survive in the marketplace of the future.

Strategic planning is a goal-oriented process of evaluation, implementation, and assessment. It relies on careful consideration of an organization's capabilities and environment and leads to priority-based resource allocation and related decisions. The vision statement is an inspiring picture of a preferred future. A vision is not bound by time; a vision represents global and continuing purposes and serves as a foundation for a system of strategic planning. For gastroenterologists, the vision statement could incorporate advancing the quality of medical care provided to patients, creating a viable long-term financial environment, or incorporating new medical knowledge and technical advances into existing organizations and operations.

Strategies are methods gastroenterologists use to achieve goals and objectives that are produced by strategic planning. A strategy is the means for transforming inputs into outputs and ultimately outcomes with the best use of resources. The steps for strategic planning for gastroenterologists are generic and simple. After defining the vision statement, the next step is to assess the current situation and identify opportunities and possible solutions. The situation analysis involves collecting information from a variety of sources, including statistics from managed care research studies, reimbursement trends, capitation trends, federal research priorities, industry priorities, professional associations, and individuals involved in the field.

The assessment of existing information forms the basis for the business plan. The business plan is a blueprint for achieving the GI organization's vision for the future. It contains detailed information on the business plans critical success factors, expected benefits and risks, financial details, and implementation schedule. Strategies for improving old business areas and entering new business areas are detailed. In developing the business plan, it is important to start with an assessment of the external environment and then relate the external forces, which are driving change, to the internal environment within the organization. The careful assessment of these external forces is used to identify market niches of opportunity.

The next step in the strategic planning process is to develop a focused implementation strategy for each component of the business plan. The importance of each component of the strategy will depend on the organization's competitive position, the market conditions, and available resources. Strategy is defined after implementation, and the strategic planner can start searching and screening all possible growth opportunities, arrange them by priority, and begin the actual implementation phase.

It is critical to be active rather than reactive during the implementation phase. In today's environment, gastroenterologists cannot passively wait for people to bring new opportunities either directly from other organizations or from business intermediaries. Gastroenterologists must actively identify target companies from directories, databases, mailing lists, trade associations, and other resources for each component of growth in the strategic plan and actively seek out representatives within those organizations. This also involves taking an aggressive attitude toward uncovering opportunities and communicating with principals rather than passively waiting for intermediaries to present situations.

One of the key determinants of success will be the ability to cultivate new business relationships. These relationships may be internal within one's organization or external within managed care organizations, academic centers, contract research organizations, pharmaceutical firms, and other sources of new service or product opportunities. Establish relationships with organizations likely to have opportunities in the future so that you have an existing dialogue before the opportunity becomes well-known. This approach is cheaper and adds more value with less risk. Gastroenterologists can significantly increase the likelihood of success in their organization by adopting an active rather than reactive development strategy through strategic planning.

After relationships are in place, the next step is to establish market awareness with your target audience. For gastroenterologists, this is accomplished through professional organization participation, publication in GI-related journals, networking with other gastroenterologists with similar business interests, and informal discussions with outside parties that have an interest in areas that you have targeted in the business plan. Prioritize the list of organizations to contact personally either through existing contacts or through networking. Use a direct-marketing campaign to inform the remainder of the organizations in your criteria of your business and your goals. Marketing brochures and other materials should be developed that address the organization's strategic plan objectives in a way that the other organization's interests are highlighted. Market awareness is not a onetime effort but an ongoing process. With a carefully designed market awareness program, gastroenterologists will be able to take advantage of new opportunities before competitors become aware of them.

The final step in the strategic planning process is the gathering of intelligence concerning those high priority organizations. The more you can learn about a target organization (e.g., company's background, key management philosophy, products, research and development goals, current financial condition, and history of licensing and partnering relationships), the better prepared you will be to discuss mutual interests. During this investigation stage, you are trying to learn of a particular organization's needs and its long-term plans while trying to identify any hidden agendas. You also need to determine if you have the potential for a business fit where value could be achieved by both parties and if an environment exists where you and the other organization could work together and adapt to each other's culture.

Strategic planning is an ongoing process. Progress towards achieving goals and objectives should be evaluated continuously, and the business plan should be critically updated on an annual basis. In today's rapidly changing health care environment, strategic planning is an invaluable tool for gastroenterologists that may even determine the difference between long-term success or failure in the field.

Managed care and a changing industry attitude towards the performance of clinical research in academic centers are creating new opportunities for gastroenterologists to participate in and profit from industry-sponsored clinical trials. The increased emphasis on the cost-effectiveness of medical care delivery has resulted in the development of clinical practice guidelines and measurement of patient outcomes as performance measures. Gastroenterologists who understand guidelines and outcomes research concepts and who demonstrate cost-effective care will be better equipped to compete for scarce resources and justify the services provided. Managed care has prompted a reexamination of the entire process of care for selected chronic diseases such as hypertension, diabetes, and inflammatory bowel disease (IBD). Disease management is a new area of opportunity for gastroenterologists that involves more specialty medical care rather than less. The remainder of this chapter focuses on four recent growth areas for gastroenterology that have surfaced as a consequence of managed care.

CLINICAL TRIALS

There is a great deal of controversy over the effect the transition to managed care will have on the pharmaceutical industry. The emerging consensus is that government financial pressure on managed care organizations to cut costs in the future may actually result in an increase in expenditure on therapeutic compounds at the cost of reduced physician time. In this scenario, a physician will be more likely to prescribe empiric drug therapy in order to reduce patient follow-up visits for chronic conditions.

The clinical trials business sector is large and growing. Today, pharmaceutical companies spend 13% of their gross sales on research and development. When worldwide pharmaceutical sales grossed $207 billion in 1993, pharmaceutical companies spent $27 billion on research and development. Clinical trials on the safety and efficacy of drugs, medical devices, or new techniques are required by the US Food and Drug Administration (FDA) for drug and device approval. Clinical trials are divided into four major phases. Phase I trials determine whether a drug or product is safe in humans and usually enroll fewer than 100 patients. Phase II trials test for efficacy in a slightly larger group of patients. Phase III and Phase IV studies often have multiple sponsors. Phase III trials are big, multicenter, randomized-controlled studies that recruit thousands of people to test the safety and efficacy of the therapy within the general population. These tests take several years to complete. Phase IV trials, which are often called outcomes studies, investigate a product once it is on the market and may look at cost-effectiveness and quality-of-life issues.

Pharmaceutical firms are concerned that clinical trials will suffer from decreased patient participation because of the spread of managed care organizations and the focus on cost competitiveness. Managed care organizations are reluctant to pay for ancillary tests and procedures performed during the course of a trial that they would not pay for otherwise. As a result, pharmaceutical firms are looking for new subjects with digestive conditions who are willing to take part in clinical trials.

Recent mergers and acquisitions in the pharmaceutical and biotechnology industry have drastically altered the corporate landscape, and perhaps nowhere have the effects been felt more than in drug company research departments. Big pharmaceutical firms are finding they cannot and should not do everything. Biotechnology firms, which are generally much smaller, are discovering the difficulties of conducting basic and applied research and manufacturing without help. These difficulties have created fertile ground for joint ventures and partnering in which the participants have some kind of financial stake (e.g., capital investment, agreements to share profits or expenses, and licensing agreements). These difficulties also have spawned a whole range of research that is completed under a pay-for-services formula. The field of contract research has grown explosively during the past decade. Independent contract research organizations (CROs) that specialize in providing generic services to pharmaceutical firms are replacing the traditional academic investigator in conducting large clinical trials for pharmaceutical companies. The principle role of the CRO is management and coordination of large multicenter trials.

The demand for physicians who are capable of serving as recruitment and study sites for industry-sponsored clinical trials is growing dramatically. Private practices trying to maintain their profit base are beginning to look at clinical trials as a source of income in their strategic plans. There are many advantages to participation in industry-sponsored trials. Participation in drug company trials may be rewarded by travel to meetings and other indirect benefits. There is the reward of academic and professional esteem, which is mainly accrued by those who write the papers and present the data. This esteem may be local, national, or international and, for some people, is a powerful motivation and reward that can be used for marketing purposes. Lastly, clinical trials can be financially lucrative if managed efficiently by gastroenterologists. Gastroenterologists who form strategic alliances with contract research organizations will be in the position to benefit from clinical trial projects that involve patients with GI conditions. Gastroenterologists interested in getting into the clinical trial business should form relationships and strategic alliances with contract resource organizations and pharmaceutical firms.

OUTCOMES RESEARCH

Another area receiving recent attention is the evolving field of outcomes research. The application of outcomes research has several domains. The most common domain has been to eval-uate therapeutics. By incorporating cost and outcomes mea-sures into the evaluation of competing therapies, researchers can determine the optimal approach based on available re-sources. Evaluation of treatment approaches should encompass pharmaceutical products, diagnostic tests, and medical proce-dures. Examples of therapeutic evaluations in gastroenterology include: 1) cost-effectiveness of misoprostol as prophylaxis against non steroidal anti-inflammatory drug–induced GI tract bleeding, 2) cost-effectiveness of preoperative testing for fecal occult blood, and 3) flexible sigmoidoscopy plus air-contrast barium enema versus colonoscopy for evaluation of sympto-matic patients without evidence of bleeding.

Another focus of outcomes research is the evaluation of clinical management strategies. These studies consider thera-peutic effectiveness and clinical decisions on the timing of in-tervention, consequences of failed treatment, patient popula-tion characteristics, and the level or degree of intervention. The evaluation of management strategies is inherently more complex than therapeutic evaluation and has a greater potential for re-ducing cost and/or increasing quality of health care. Examples of outcomes research involving GI management strategies include: 1) initial endoscopy or empirical therapy with or without testing for *Helicobacter pylori* for dyspepsia, 2) treatment of chronic type B and C hepatitis with interferon-α, and 3) endoscopic retro-grade cannulation of pancreatic duct (ERCP) versus surgery for the treatment of malignant biliary obstruction.

A second domain of outcomes research that is becoming increasingly important is the evaluation of institutional per-formance. Evaluating institutional performance involves the application of outcomes research to an entire institution by sampling outcomes of the client population. The measurement of institutional performance can be conducted internally to identify areas of potential improvement or externally to compare organizations to one another. As market pressures force the containment and reduction of costs, employers will use outcomes data to evaluate employee health plans and patients will use outcomes data to select among competing plans. The practicing gastroenterologist who understands the concepts of outcomes research and is able to demonstrate cost-effective treatment will be better able to compete in the managed care environment. Several options are available to assist private practice gastroenterologists in measuring outcomes. These include working with hospital-based resource groups, tracking endoscopic procedures, networking with other members of endoscopic database groups, measuring outcomes in the office setting, and working with managed care organizations or other payers. Ideally, outcomes should be linked across all patient visits, including inpatient and outpatient.

Hospitals are becoming more aware of the need to document patient outcomes. Many have already critically evaluated the quality of care delivered to their patients and have established critical care pathways for common admitting diagnoses. This enables hospitals to compare their outcomes with national benchmark data and anonymously with other providers who use the same hospital. Admissions for digestive disorders such as GI hemorrhage, IBD, or diverticulitis are particularly suited for this approach. Working within the context of the hospital, outcomes (e.g., mortality, complication rates, length of stay, resource utilization, and, in some cases, patient satisfaction) are accessible to individual providers who may be too busy to compile the data themselves.

More data are needed to measure immediate, short-term, and long-term outcomes in community practice. Immediate outcomes should focus on technical success such as the frequency with which the cecum is reached during colonoscopy and procedure-related complications and patient satisfaction using standardized definitions. Short-term outcomes should include follow-up of complications and functional success (i.e., an improvement in functional status). Long-term outcomes should include quality-of-life assessment. The benefits of collecting these data are obvious: consumer demand. If a gastroenterology practice cannot provide this information, it will be difficult for that practice to compete with providers who do. The amount of work involved is the limitation of these types of studies. Either physician or support personnel time is required to enter, access, and analyze the data. The increased availability of support among larger office-based practices, however, makes it possible to undertake such studies.

Large scale outcomes research is best carried out by a multidisciplinary team of investigators. Such a team would include gastroenterologists and individuals with expertise in survey research, health services research, biostatistics, decision analysis, and economics and pharmacoeconomics. Although training is required to design and conduct valid outcomes studies, outcomes data are best collected at the clinical level by physicians and their staff. The ideal data source for outcomes research is prospective, protocol-driven, data collection programs that are based on refined research questions.

The trend towards increasing evaluation of digestive disease treatments can be expected to continue as long as the resultant economic savings and improved quality of life exceed the cost of conducting those studies. Outcomes research is currently an expensive undertaking. The longitudinal follow-up of patient populations requires dedicated study coordinators, data managers, medical coders, and other support personnel. However, this situation is improving because of new advances in integrated computer and telecommunications systems specifically designed for the collection of point-of-contact medical care utilization and quality of life information. Technology that has already been proven in other fields (e.g., electronic banking) could dramatically reduce the cost of collecting economic and outcomes data to the point where it could be incorporated seamlessly into the day-to-day operations of a provider organization. As the cost of conducting outcomes research goes down, the volume of studies conducted will increase.

In the past, outcomes research has been financed primarily by federal sources, but this too is changing. Large health care provider organizations and their consultants are setting up internal outcomes assessment units to evaluate and optimize in-house operations. The pharmaceutical industry is establishing and expanding pharmacoeconomic units and incorporating health-related quality of life (HRQOL) measures in regulatory trials of new products.

Outcomes research in digestive diseases is an important tool for evaluation treatment strategies and determining the best approach for a given patient. Outcomes studies will be used by policy makers, administrators, managers, and other non-physicians to select treatment strategies that maximize quality and minimize cost. These studies will include quality of life as a principal determinant of efficacy. In addition, severity-adjusted outcomes data will be used to measure institutional performance and compare the structure and process of health care in different settings. Gastroenterologists must be trained in developing well-designed outcomes assessment data. Also, gastroenterologists must be equally well-trained in evaluating such data, and they must develop sufficient expertise so that they can influence decisions regarding managed care in GI disorders.

CLINICAL PRACTICE GUIDELINES

Clinical practice guidelines are increasingly considered by professional bodies, governments, and consumer organizations as a means of improving health outcomes and quality of patient care. Clinical practice guidelines are especially important in gastroenterology where clinical decision making plays a large role in cost-effective outcomes. Clinical practice guidelines are not a new phenomenon. Informal standards have always been adhered to by any group of physicians within a particular institution. Guidelines have existed in clinical practice for decades and were referred to as practice guidelines, practice policies, clinical policies, protocols, clinical algorithms, position statements, and principles of practice.

In the past, guidelines were developed by single experts or by a panel of experts. The expert opinion guidelines were subject to bias because of the following: the composition of the expert opinion guideline was not systematic, the panels composing the expert opinion guideline often entirely consisted of academic tertiary care specialists, and the process for creating the expert opinion guideline was not formalized or documented.

Today, the process of guideline development is highly structured. Guidelines are developed by a panel of multidisciplinary experts using replicable processes. Guidelines are supplemented by a systematic literature review and meta-analyses to ensure an evidence-based approach. In the United States, the implementation of guidelines is increasingly being subjected to either retrospective or prospective evaluation to establish impact on health care. These changes to the guideline development and implementation process are designed to improve usefulness, acceptability, reliability, validity, and predictability.

Several key attributes determine the quality of a clinical practice guideline. The first attribute is validity; the guideline should be based on strong scientific evidence. A practice guideline must also be reliable and reproducible. The users of the guidelines should reach the same decisions over time and across different user groups, and similar guidelines should emerge if the guideline's development process were replicated. Guidelines must be outcomes-focused to ensure they achieve desired results. They should also allow for incorporation of patient preferences and differences in organizational capabilities, resources, and other similar factors.

Implementation of guidelines is highly variable. Only recently health care organizations received direction on optimal processes for the development and implementation of clinical guidelines through the work of the US Agency for Health Care Policy and Research and associated industry organizations.

Another new initiative in health care improvement processes is the critical pathway. Critical pathways, clinical pathways, care maps, and care plans are documented plans of expected clinical management where the critical treatments and interventions are identified and sequenced along a time line. Pathways pick up where guidelines often leave off; they are invoked after the decision to apply a particular procedure has been made, and they typically concern the specific details of care. The intention of the pathway is to chart a clinical process from start to finish and sometimes beyond, including the time anticipated to complete key activities in the process. Some pathways include expected outcomes at each stage of the process. The critical pathway is usually multidisciplinary and divided into key functional areas such as consultations, tests, treatments, medications, diet, activity, patient education, and discharge planning. Once implemented, each patient may be tracked to assess progress and pinpoint areas of variation from the map that may require further discussion or action.

Substantial roles currently exist for the development and evaluation of guidelines in gastroenterology. The practicing gastroenterologist, acting as a consultant to management and accounting firms, is able to provide the scientific expertise needed to conduct large scale studies of the cost-effectiveness of guidelines. Gastroenterologists are doing much work in the development and evaluation of critical pathways.

DISEASE MANAGEMENT

The managed care movement has prompted policy makers to rethink many aspects of our health care system. One interesting area of emphasis is disease management for certain chronic conditions such as hypertension, diabetes, and IBD.

Efforts have been made over the previous 30 years to evaluate and improve the cost-effectiveness and quality of health care in the United States. Despite these efforts, health care costs have risen from 4% to 14% of the gross domestic national product. During the same period, the United States has ranked low on the list of industrialized nations in important health care indicators such as infant mortality. Research on the appropriateness of medical care in the United States indicates as much as 25% of medical care is unjustified and as many as 25% of all hospital deaths may be preventable. With respect to access to care, more than 39 million people or 16% of the population currently lack medical insurance. These statistics highlight systematic flaws in the structure, process, and outcomes of health care delivery in the United States. Although managed care is creating new competition among providers, insurers, and employers, the impact of managed care on the quality of care remains poorly measured and highly controversial.

Recently, disease management has been proposed as a means of controlling or reducing costs while simultaneously increasing the overall quality of care. Disease management involves a rethinking and realigning of the structure and process of health care from a systems' perspective. The disease management model allows the creation of structure and process characteristics that are targeted at a specific medical condition. The disease management model is best suited for chronic diseases that have a high cumulative cost and outcome impact during the lifetime of a patient.

In the US health care system, the traditional unit of analysis for evaluation of cost of care is the institutional department, the practitioner, the procedure, the medication, or some other directly identifiable resource unit. As a result, a highly fragmented system of accounting and measuring has evolved where each component of the system is managed separately often by individuals with competing motivations and incentives. As an example, a hospital pharmacy department may institute a program to reduce medication costs by establishing guidelines that limit and restrict the prescription of high cost medicines. Paradoxically, such programs may have just the opposite effect on system-wide costs. A University of Utah study charted the cost of treating 24,000 patients compared to the cost of treating patients at HMOs with and without formulary restrictions. The study found that patients with a limited drug choice made more visits, including emergency room visits and hospitalizations, during the course of a year. Those patients also had higher yearly drug costs and numbers of prescriptions. The study concluded patient cost was higher in HMOs with formulary restriction because the patients did not always get the drug they needed. The study estimated the cost of treatment could be cut by 50% through the use of more appropriate therapy. The disease management model involves application of a systems' approach to the appropriate treatment. The disease itself is the unit of analysis in disease management.

Advances in the structure and process of care can be more readily identified, evaluated, and incorporated into an integrated system of care by focusing the evaluation process on the disease. In a disease management setting, the provider organization would ideally contract with managed care providers to capitate 100% of the health care costs for a patient with a chronic condition during a multiyear period. Disease management organizations would employ medical subspecialists who would provide chronic specialty care and evaluate the primary care needs for enrollees. Since financial performance of the disease management organization would be determined by long-term containment and reduction in patient care costs, incentive would exist for investment of capital to identify cost-effective outcome improvements.

The concept of continuous quality improvement (CQI) is directly applicable to disease management organizations. CQI concepts and applications are designed to allow fragmented health care delivery organizations to overcome some of the traditional barriers to quality improvement. CQI has a systems' approach to the prospective identification of quality deficiencies and implementation of quality-enhancing solutions. The same techniques can be used by disease management organizations to achieve continuous quality improvement.

The ideal disease management program has a structure, process standards, and outcome measures designed to minimize long-term program costs and maximize short-term and long-term patient outcomes. Maximizing patient outcomes is achieved by ensuring all necessary health care for a patient population is provided in a timely manner. Minimizing cost is achieved by ensuring there is no waste or unnecessary care provided and the appropriate level of intervention is applied at all times. Both goals are achieved through the continuous monitoring and evaluation of the causal association between process and outcome. Successful disease management organizations have structure, process, and outcome characteristics that support the achievement of these goals.

The ideal structure of a disease management program for chronic disease differs in several important respects from traditional health care delivery structures in the United States.

Characteristics that optimize the structure of disease management delivery include an outpatient-based setting, staff diversity, mechanisms for continuous monitoring of the patient-client base outside of the clinic setting, and a high level of information technology infrastructure. The chronic disease management organization should become a distributed matrix management model that allows wide geographic distribution of health care services; the management organization would be interconnected through an information linkage. The facility should be outpatient-based to reflect the cost savings and outcome improvements achievable through early intervention strategies. Although initial contact centers would be distributed, diagnostic and therapeutic procedures could be batch-scheduled and performed at central locations for more efficient use of expensive personnel and equipment. Results would be transmitted electronically between initial contact sites and central procedure centers.

The management organization and personnel should also reflect a matrix model. In disease management, the notion of practitioner takes on an expanded definition that includes physicians, nurses, and other medical care staff and extends to case managers, screening and medical triage personnel, and health care support professionals. The types of practitioners include cognitive behavioral therapists, alternative or complementary treatment providers, and educators. In the chronic disease management model, the efficient use of personnel resources requires a hierarchy of expertise. The goal is to avoid to overuse or underutilize the level of practitioner intervention for a given patient situation. The front line of the practitioner-patient interaction could be a case manager who is specifically trained to make triage decisions regarding patient intervention or referral. The use of a patient educator early in the treatment process could greatly reduce the amount of subspecialist time spent explaining lay disease principles to patients and result in cost savings that do not impact quality of care.

A high level of information infrastructure is required to support disease management programs. Monitoring information into database systems that can provide decision support is required. Automated medical records can be used to eliminate redundancy and waste. Automated patient contact and monitoring systems can provide seamless collection of severity and risk factor data. Automated practice guidelines and practice criteria can be used to reduce variation and increase quality assurance. Decision models, artificial intelligence diagnostic programs, neural network models, influence diagrams, and other tools would be used to provide decision support. The technology exists today to provide for all these needs, however, it has been poorly applied to the medical care setting.

Process is a dynamic entity that constantly changes as new knowledge is acquired about the disease, patient, and outcome of treatment strategies. The evaluation of process must also be a dynamic and continuous undertaking. Establishment of practice guidelines and treatment protocols is the core of the continuous quality and cost-effectiveness (profit) improvement program for the organization. Methods currently exist for measuring appropriateness. Formal systems of review and evaluation should be implemented and tracked using the infrastructure of the information systems. Current guidelines should be evaluated and adopted. Efforts should be made towards implementing systems of continuous guideline improvement to reflect changes in diagnostic and treatment technologies as they are introduced into the marketplace and to reflect new advances in medical knowledge. The standard classification of treatment into appropriate, equivocal, and inappropriate can be used prospectively to integrate clinical trials directly into the treatment setting. Any treatment that is considered equivocal would be subjected to randomized clinical-effectiveness trials.

Two driving factors that define the success of a disease management process are early detection and timeliness. Early detection can be achieved in a number of ways. One is increased monitoring. Patients may be required to submit to routine monitoring of their disease status in order to chart severity of disease over time. Another method to detect problems earlier is patient education. Patients who are taught to recognize warning signs of increasing disease severity can seek more timely and appropriate intervention. In evaluating timeliness, developers of a disease management program may determine during evaluation of traditional physical barriers to patient access (e.g., transportation and work schedule conflicts) that it is cost-effective to pay these external costs if it results in reduced medical costs and outcomes. Taking this concept one step further, they may find it cost-effective to have practitioners make house calls on patients if time lines result in lower medical costs.

Evaluation of outcome in cost, patient satisfaction, quality of life, and other parameters in the disease management model provides the empirical data required for the continuous refinement and improvement of process of care. This forms a continuous quality improvement loop that drives the cost-effectiveness of the organization. Outcomes data should be collected on a routine basis to identify patients at risk of using medical resources; these patients may be candidates for early intervention protocols.

A great deal of research has been published during the previous 20 years on methods for outcome measurement. These tools should be used and adapted by disease management organizations to track patient outcomes and measure severity of illness over time. Longitudinal tracking of data is required in outcomes assessment to measure change in outcome so that the cause and effect relationship between process and outcome can be investigated. Rules of ensuring compliance with collection of outcomes data should be built into the health care plan either as a contractual requirement between patient and provider organization or through financial incentives for providing outcomes data.

No clear answer exists to the question of who should establish and run disease management programs, which is perhaps a reflection of the fragmented structure of the current US health care system. Existing organizations that could be considered include academic institutions, pharmaceutical companies, specialty provider groups, and managed care organizations. There are examples of academic centers of excellence that have established comprehensive disease management programs in the fee-for-service setting.

Academic programs may be optimized for maximizing patient outcomes, however, mechanisms for evaluating cost-effectiveness are not a part of these centers. Excellence in many academic institutions translates to having access to the latest and most expensive treatment technologies. The translation of the use of these technologies into improved outcomes is not well-documented. In addition, academic centers traditionally do not have the business management expertise, the capital investment structure, or ability to make the commitment of capital for long-range gains. Thus, some of the structure and process expertise required for high quality disease management organization exists in academic centers. Financial incentives and mechanisms for measuring cost-effectiveness do not currently exist.

Pharmaceutical companies are logical candidates for entering the disease management business, especially when treatment for a disease is highly dependent on patented therapeutics. Pharmaceutical companies in the managed care environment are searching for ways to expand their product offering in response to competitive downward negotiation of purchase price from HMOs and purchasing cooperatives. Under this scenario, a pharmaceutical firm would invest capital to start-up a disease management program for a specific chronic condition. The pharmaceutical company would then establish a pilot program for a specific geographic area using the business planning principles discussed earlier. After entering the disease management business, a pharmaceutical company will try to find ways of decreasing the use of its own medications as part of cost-effectiveness evaluation under a disease management scenario. This may create conflicts between sales and disease management divisions within the same company.

Specialty medical care groups have some of the business structure required to set up disease management programs. For example, the four largest independent practice associations (IPA) in the San Francisco Bay Area are currently under merger negotiations. An IPA-based organization could be a potential candidate for establishing disease management programs in large urban centers

DISEASE MANAGEMENT PROGRAM FOR INFLAMMATORY BOWEL DISEASE

As an illustration of the role of the gastroenterologist in GI disease management, we consider IBD. The design of a disease management program for IBD should become a business plan that includes standard components including market assessment, evaluation of current epidemiology and patient care practices, program design, and a financial plan and risk assessment. Market Assessment Inflammatory Bowel Disease is a chronic condition of obscure etiology that most often begins in the second and third decade of life. There is no known cure for the condition other than surgical resection of the bowel. Patients often live with IBD symptoms for the remainder of life. IBD currently affects between 0.1 and 0.2% of the US population or as many as 500,000 individuals. Incidence rates for IBD have been estimated at 10.7 per 100,000 population per year. The condition is associated with significant morbidity and cost and resulted in approximately 700,000 physician visits and 100,000 hospital discharges occurring in the United States each year. The estimated annual cost of treating IBD is estimated at 820 million dollars per year.

The relative rarity of the disease suggests that an effective disease management approach may only be feasible in large urban centers because of the economy-of-scale considerations. For example, the 1990 population estimate for Los Angeles County is 8,863,164 persons or 3.56% of the total US population. By extrapolation, this geographic region should contain between 8,863 to 17,726 persons with IBD and the annual incidence rate would be approximately 150 new cases per year. An assessment should be made of the minimum population needed to achieve required economy-of-scale for a disease management program.

There are a number of well-known but poorly understood risk factors for increased severity of illness. These include: urban versus rural residence, ethnicity, familial aggregation, diet, smoking (protective), alcohol and coffee consumption, and the use of oral contraceptives. Patients with IBD may have an increased risk for colon cancer, and complications of IBD include ankylosing spondylitis and sclerosing cholangitis. Current treatment practices are centered on control of symptoms through anti-inflammatory medication with surgical options for severe disease. Laboratory monitoring of blood and serum chemistry levels is often used to determine medication dosing. Diagnostic procedures including colonoscopy, barium enema, and sigmoidoscopy are used frequently in outpatient and inpatient settings. Hospitalization is often required for disease flare-ups, and emergent admissions occur especially in the underinsured populations with IBD.

Design elements that may be incorporated into a high quality, cost-effective disease management program for IBD include a patient monitoring system, an early intervention system, patient involvement and empowerment, and appropriate level of personnel expertise.

Systematic patient monitoring may be achieved through computerized information systems that are combined with the use of case managers as the primary point of contact for all patients. Information systems and a comprehensive patient management database would be developed to track patient appointments and schedule prospective routine follow-up information for each patient. In addition, monitoring systems would track parameters such as individual risk factors, symptom and flare-up history, medication and treatment compliance, level of patient knowledge, and transcripts of all patient contacts. Tickler reports and other information resources would be provided to case managers to prompt required prospective actions.

Monitoring would also include outcomes data with emphasis placed on collecting uniform information on a periodic basis. Systematic tracking of patient functional status and health-related quality of life would be instituted for all patients using the validated IBD health status questionnaire, which includes the Crohn's and colitis disease activity index, the generic Short Form-36 question quality of life questionnaire (SF-36) questionnaire, and the Group Health Association of America's consumer satisfaction survey. The goal of the monitoring component would be to provide a proactive rather that a reactive capability for identifying and meeting routine patient medical care needs for patients with IBD. Ongoing evaluation of the effectiveness of the system in cost and outcomes would be conducted using continuous quality improvement methods.

Early intervention protocols and algorithms that use the monitoring database would be put in place. Risk factor modeling and other statistical techniques would be used to tailor programmed patient intervention to a particular patient based on his or her individual disease and socio-demographic characteristics. Decision analysis, neural networking, and other predictive techniques would be evaluated for ability to reduce cost and improve outcomes. The use of computer-assisted telephone symptom recording protocols and other data collection tools currently being used in clinical trials may be useful in tracking daily variation in patient symptoms, which could be used to further refine staging systems. The goal of the early intervention program would be to convert inpatient episodes into outpatient episodes through early detection and treatment.

In the traditional US medical care setting, patient health care programs are not considered a part of the medical care delivery process. The advantage of the disease management approach for a chronic condition such as IBD is that nonmedical patient interventions that are cost-effective can be easily incorporated into the overall patient care program. Often such programs can reduce cost and improve outcomes and patient satisfaction. These interventions would include patient education on topics such as how to discriminate between benign symptoms and serious symptoms, nutritional modulation of symptoms, patient support groups to reduce psychosocial stress that can exacerbate IBD symptoms, and training in self-medication and self-dosing of common medications. Patient education programs focusing on cognitive-behavioral education may be cost-effective when they result in early recognition. Medical treatments could be replaced with nonmedical intervention for areas such as pain reduction and stress control.

Another advantage of the disease management approach is that alternatives to the traditional patient-physician relationship can be explored. Personnel inefficiencies can be optimized by diversifying staff in a disease management organization. For example, the most time-efficient use of a physician or subspecialist is in diagnosing and developing treatment plans for patients with IBD. If psychosocial intervention, nutritional evaluation, or other ancillary services are required, they are best handled by other lesser and more cost-effective personnel. The trained case manager who serves as the initial point of patient contact could answer simple questions, address patient concerns, and triage all contacts and in this way decrease inappropriate use of expensive subspecialist time.

The national annual summary data for the direct costs of patients with IBD in the United States are 537.7 million dollars for inpatient services, 30.3 million dollars for outpatient care, and 20.5 million dollars for prescription drugs. The current ratio of outpatient visits to inpatient admissions for IBD are 7:1; the yearly risk of an outpatient visit is 33% per year, and the annual risk of an inpatient admission is 4.3%. The high dependence on medication combined with the financial consequences of inadequately monitored disease symptoms make IBD an excellent candidate for a disease management program. Financial goals of the program would center on the elimination of emergent care and a decrease in rates of surgical intervention and inpatient admissions. The technical approach to achieving these goals would involve development of a specialized patient-monitoring structure and process protocols. An investment would be made in outpatient care and patient outreach programs that would be offset by reduced inpatient and surgical costs. A successful disease management program would require long-term financial commitment and start-up cost that would be recouped in the out years of the program. Negotiation of patient management contracts should cover 5- to 10-year periods, if feasible. The financial risks of undertaking such a program include unforeseen short-term changes in the epidemiology of the disease, the inability to shift inpatient care to the outpatient setting, and the failure to reach the economy-of-scale required to design and implement a patient-monitoring structure and process standards.

It is unclear at this point whether disease management will become a wave of the future or merely a whim of the present. Patients, as increasingly informed consumers of heath care services, are also interested in cost-effectiveness and outcomes. Employers and insurers will be interested in disease management programs from a cost standpoint. The commercial incentive for investing in disease management exists mainly because of the inefficiencies embedded in our current health care system for the treatment of certain chronic disease.

CONCLUSIONS

The rapid transition from fee-for-service to managed care in the United States has created an environment of unprecedented change and uncertainty for the gastroenterologist. The move to managed care is resulting in an increased scrutiny and the decreased utilization of subspecialty services. However, it is not clear whether this trend is cost-effective and in the best interest of the patient.

Strategic planning is a tool that can be used by gastroenterologists to manage change. Managed care brings along with it new opportunities for growth as well as constraints on subspecialty medicine. The successful gastroenterologist of the future can use strategic planning to take advantage of new opportunities to minimize the negative impact of managed care and take advantage of new areas of potential growth.

SUGGESTED READINGS

Eisenberg DM, Kessler RC, Foster C, et al. Unconventional medicine in the United States. Prevalence, costs, and patterns of use. N Engl J Med 1993;328:246–252. (This is a landmark survey on the use of alternative therapies.)

Gitnick G, Rothenberg F, Weiner J. The business of medicine. New York: Elsevier, 1991. (This compendium of business information for the private practitioner has many references specific to the gastroenterologist.)

Horn SD. Unintended consequences of drug formularies. American Journal of Health-System Pharmacy, 1996 Sep 15, 53(18):2204–2206. (This report gives excellent examples of why a systems approach must be used when implementing cost-effectiveness measures in an HMO setting.)

Marwick C. Another health care idea: disease management [news]. JAMA 1995;274:1416–1417.

Mechanic. The impact of managed care on clinical research: a preliminary investigation: final report. PHS Contract No. 282–92-0041. Washington, DC: US Government Printing Office, January 1996. (One of the first government reports that examines the relationship between traditional clinical research and the expected impact of the managed care shift on the ability to perform government- and industry-sponsored clinical studies.)

Sandler R, et al. A primer on outcomes research for the gastroenterologist: report of the American Gastroenterological Association task force on outcomes research. Gastroenterology 1995;109: 302–306. (This primer explains outcomes research and why it is important for the practice of gastroenterology.)

US Department of Health and Human Services, Public Health Service. National Institutes of Health, National Institute of Diabetes and Digestive and Kidney Diseases. Digestive diseases in the United States: epidemiology and impact. NIH publication 94–1447. Washington, DC: US Government Printing Office, 1994. (This is another government report that serves as the bible of digestive disease epidemiology and economic impact. An invaluable resource for description of disease trends; this resource is divided by GI disorder and discusses the future treatment for digestive disorders.)

Chapter Two

PROTON PUMP INHIBITORS: WHEN TO ADMINISTER AND WHEN NOT TO ADMINISTER

Melvyn G. Korman, MD, and Fiona B. Nicholson, MD

INTRODUCTION

Acid secretion by the stomach has been researched for many decades. Not only have clinicians attempted to understand how the stomach secretes acid, but they have sought effective ways of treating common disorders associated with acid secretion such as peptic ulcer disease or reflux esophagitis.

Gastric acid is secreted from the parietal cell of the stomach. The enzyme responsible for secreting gastric acid is the H^+,K^+-adenosinetriphosphatase (ATPase), which is the gastric acid pump. This proton pump is found in large quantities only in the parietal cell.

Treatment of acid-related disorders during the previous 20 years has been revolutionized by the development of two new classes of drugs: histamine receptor antagonists (H_2RAs) and proton pump inhibitors (PPIs). Both drugs affect the parietal cell and reduce acid secretion. However, the mechanisms of action in H_2RAs and PPIs are quite distinct, and H_2RA and PPI treatment differ in their therapeutic value and application.

The intragastric pH level should be maintained at or above 3 for most of a 24-hour period for effective healing in patients with ulcer-related disease. The pH level should be more than 4 for effective healing in patients with gastroesophageal reflux disease (GERD), while the pH levels for effective treatment of *Helicobacter pylori* infection may need to be even higher since the potency of antibiotics is increased with higher intragastric pH levels. The question remains as to how such levels of intragastric pH can be reliably achieved.

Available treatment modalities for the reduction of gastric acid secretion in patients include antacids, H_2RAs, and PPIs. Antacids produce rapid short-lived symptom relief by neutralizing acid already secreted into the stomach. However, antacids require frequent large doses, and, although occasional use of antacids may relieve minor symptoms, their use as proven therapeutic agents seems impractical. Antacid treatment for acid-related disease is outdated.

Direct inhibition of acid secretion by the parietal cell is the current treatment of choice. The first clinical studies of H_2RA treatment approximately 20 years ago changed the management of patients with acid-related disorders, particularly peptic ulcer disease. The initial H_2RA treatment was cimetidine and was soon followed by ranitidine and more recently, famotidine, nizatidine, and roxatidine. The introduction of these drugs significantly reduced the number of operations and duration of illness in patients and shortened hospital stays.

Despite the superior efficacy of H_2RA treatment to traditional antacid therapy, H_2RA treatment has significant shortcomings. H_2RA treatment is not effective therapy for all acute and chronic acid-related diseases, in particular ulcerative GERD and refractory peptic ulcer. Despite prolonged therapy with H_2RA, significant numbers of patients with peptic ulcer disease remain symptomatic and in approximately 10% of patients ulces do not heal. This is particularly true for patients with gastric ulcer disease, and surgery remains the only option for this patient group.

The introduction of PPI treatment solved many of these difficulties. The first introduced PPI was omeprazole, which was followed by lanzoprazole and pantoprazole, all of which are substituted benzimidazoles. PPI treatment is effective in reducing gastric acid secretion and managing most acid-related disorders. The efficacy and widespread availability of PPI treatment now poses the following questions for the clinician: when should a PPI be administered, and when is it appropriate to use alternative therapy? This chapter provides information to help the clinician answer this question.

GOALS OF PATIENT THERAPY FOR ACID-RELATED DISORDERS

The goals of therapy in patients with acid-related disorders are the following: to provide rapid symptom relief and prompt ulcer healing, avoid complications, and prevent recurrence. Such goals are most easily achieved by inhibition of acid secretion, but the increasing awareness of the need to effectively treat *H. pylori* infection in patients holds great promise for the cure of peptic ulcer disease.

All patients with acid-related disorders respond rapidly to successful suppression of gastric acid secretion. However, the extent to which gastric pH levels must be elevated in order to obtain optimal symptom relief and healing in patients with ulceration is different in the therapy of reflux esophagitis and peptic ulcer disease. The relationship of acid secretion control to healing rates in patients with duodenal ulcer disease or reflux esophagitis has been examined through meta-analysis. Healing rates were compared to the expected 24-hour values of intragastric acidity so that the pH level and the duration that the pH level is maintained can be directly equated with optimal healing rates. If the target pH of 3 is achieved for at least 17 hours out of a 24-hour period, then the minimal healing rate for duodenal ulcer is achieved. However, in reflux esophagitis the optimal healing rate requires a target pH level of 4 for 16 hours in a 24-hour period. Thus, greater acid inhibition is required for the treatment of esophagitis than for duodenal ulcer disease. These results indicate H_2RA treatment will fail to achieve the target pH level for a sufficient period of time to provide optimal healing in patients with duodenal ulcer disease and fall short of the target pH level for healing in patients with ulcerative reflux esophagitis. In contrast, PPI treatment achieves the target pH level for sufficient time to provide optimal healing in patients with duodenal ulcer disease and ulcerative esophagitis. The target intragastric pH level needed is approximately 5 for most of a 24-hour period for effective antibiotic treatment of H. *pylori* infection. Thus, management of H. *pylori* infection in patients requires profound gastric acid inhibition and seems to demand PPI treatment rather than H_2RA treatment.

MAJOR DIFFERENCES BETWEEN HISTAMINE RECEPTOR ANTAGONISTS AND PROTON PUMP INHIBITORS

H_2RA treatment inhibits gastric acid secretion by competing with histamine for the H_2 receptor on the parietal cell. PPI treatment inhibits gastric acid by blocking the H^+,K^+-ATPase, which is the acid secretory pump embedded within the canalicular membrane. This pump is the final step in the acid secretory process. These different modes of action signal marked differences in the pharmacology of H_2RA and PPI treatment. At routine doses, PPI treatment induces more profound acid inhibition than H_2RA treatment. Long-term maintenance of acid inhibition occurs with PPI treatment, whereas the acid inhibitory effect of H_2RA treatment fades or patients' develop a tolerance during prolonged or high dose therapy.

H_2RA treatment is effective only while patient plasma levels exceed those required to compete with endogenous histamine at the H_2 receptor site on the parietal cell. Since the plasma half-life of H_2RA is approximately 2 hours, the duration of action is short. Therefore multiple doses of H_2RA treatment may be necessary, and H_2RA treatment is often required at high doses. This limits the usefulness of H_2RA treatment especially when powerful acid suppression is required. PPI treatment inhibits the final step of acid secretion at the H^+K^+-ATPase regardless of the stimulus. Whilst H_2RA treatment is short-acting, PPI treatment has a longer duration of action, which is often more than 24 hours. PPI treatment has a short plasma half-life but a prolonged effect because restoration of gastric acid secretion requires synthesis of new PPIs. These differences in mode of action introduce the concept that PPI treatment is superior to H$_2$RA treatment in lowering gastric acid secretion.

SAFETY PROFILE OF HISTAMINE RECEPTOR ANTAGONIST AND PROTON PUMP INHIBITOR TREATMENT

SIDE EFFECT PROFILE

H$_2$RA and PPI treatment is well tolerated by patients. Marketing studies have shown H$_2$RAs are probably amongst the safest available class of drugs. Minor side effects include gastrointestinal upset, headache, and skin rash. Major side effects include gynecomastia and confusional states in the elderly, but these are quite rare. PPIs have similar minor adverse effects, which include constipation, diarrhea, vomiting, peripheral edema, and non-specific headache and migraine. The incidence of serious adverse effects is less than 1% and include isolated reports of skin rash, gynecomastia, hemolytic anaemia, and rhabdomyolysis. It is rare that side effects require cessation or alteration of H$_2$RA or PPI treatment.

There is a theoretical risk of gastric malignancy, particularly carcinoid tumors, in patients with long-term marked acid suppression. The risk is related to an increase in gastrin levels associated with the decrease in acid secretion. Long-term studies of PPI treatment show a moderate increase in gastrin levels and no evidence of gastric enterochromaffin-like cell hyperplasia, dysplasia, or metaplasia. Long-term therapy with a PPI is safe, but follow-up studies of patients for more than 15 years have not occurred.

DRUG INTERACTIONS

Cimetidine, the original H$_2$RA, has significant interaction with the cytochrome P450 enzyme system in the liver. Cimetidine metabolically and clinically interacts with drugs metabolized by the cytochrome P450 enzyme system because of this effect. These drugs include warfarin, theophylline, and digoxin. These drug interactions are less with the newer H$_2$RAs such as famotidine.

The first PPI, omeprazole, also interacts with a specific enzyme in the cytochrome P450 system. This effect is of dubious clinical significance. The newer PPIs do not share this interaction and therefore can be administered to patients taking low dose oral contraceptive pills or other drugs such as diazepam, carbamazepine, or warfarin if there are clinical concerns regarding drug interactions.

THERAPY OF ACID-RELATED DISORDERS

PEPTIC ULCER DISEASE

PPI treatment in recommended doses induces much faster ulcer healing and symptom relief than H$_2$RA treatment. The major differences between these two classes of antisecretory drugs is obvious in the early days of treatment and less marked at the end of a 4-week treatment period. Endoscopy at 2 weeks rather than at 4 weeks shows a greater difference in favor of PPI treatment. Studies show PPI treatment is effective in patients with ulcers resistant to prolonged high doses of H$_2$RAs. Ulcer pain is related to the presence of acid. Although H$_2$RA treatment provides a great advance and relieves pain in most patients within hours or days, mild symptoms persist in a considerable number of patients. In such patients, PPI administration relieves the pain within 24 to 48 hours. In general, pain relief is approximately twice as fast with PPI treatment than with H_2RA treatment. Approximately 10% of patients with peptic ulcer disease are not effectively managed with H_2RA treatment even when given in high doses and for a prolonged period of time. Yet, PPI treatment is effective in nearly all patient's with H_2RA-resistant ulcers and even peptic ulcers refractory to major gastric surgery. Such ulcers remain healed during maintenance therapy with a PPI.

DUODENAL ULCER DISEASE

Effective inhibition of gastric acid secretion through H_2RA treatment transformed the management of duodenal ulcer disease. Healing rates of patients with duodenal ulcers undergoing H_2RA treatment are reported at 50%, 78%, and 92% after 2, 4, or 8 weeks of treatment, respectively. PPIs heal ulcers in approximately 80% of duodenal ulcer patients after 2 weeks of treatment and heal 100% of ulcers after 4 weeks of treatment. Numerous multicenter double-blind studies suggest that PPI treatment provides faster symptom relief and is more effective earlier than H_2RA treatment. Meta-analysis shows a therapeutic gain of at least 30% in the first 2 weeks for patients undergoing PPI treatment compared to H_2RA treatment. Higher doses of PPIs provide additional benefit when risk factors are present. Patient risk factors that may indicate a need for higher doses or longer treatment regimens include poor response to H_2RA therapy, large ulcers, heavy smoking, and a young age of disease onset. Most duodenal ulcers will relapse upon cessation of acid suppression. Thus, maintenance therapy with H_2RAs became routine in the 1980s. Relapse rates after cessation of H_2RA or PPI therapy are similar. Deciding whether to prescribe H$_2$RA or PPI treatment as maintenance therapy depends upon the patient's symptomatic response. Most patients with duodenal ulcers are symptom-free on long-term H$_2$RA treatment.

The establishment of the causative role of *H. pylori* infection in duodenal ulcer disease has rapidly changed the role of gastric acid suppression in patients. Most patients with duodenal ulcers in the late 1980s required either intermittent or continuous maintenance therapy with H$_2$RA treatment. It seemed reasonable to reserve PPI treatment for patients whose ulcers were ineffectively treated or whose symptoms were not controlled with either short- or long-term maintenance therapy with H$_2$RAs. It has now been shown effective treatment of *H. pylori* infection in patients results in fewer ulcer recurrences, thus removing the need for maintenance therapy with either H$_2$RA or PPI treatment. Effective treatment of *H. pylori* infection should be offered to all patients with duodenal ulcers, to patients with complications, and to patients who are currently on long-term antisecretory therapy. Cure can be expected in most patients.

GASTRIC ULCER DISEASE

The pathogenesis of gastric ulcer disease is similar to that of duodenal ulcer disease. In both disorders, the formation of ulcers depends on the presence of acid and pepsin in gastric juice. *H. pylori* infection in patients also causes gastric ulcer disease. In addition, the use of non-steroidal anti-inflammatory drugs (NSAIDs) and aspirin contributes significantly to the pathogenesis of gastric ulcer disease in those patients in whom *H. pylori* infection does not appear to be the cause. Standard therapy for this disease was also H$_2$RA treatment, although required treatment duration was often longer than treatment for duodenal ulcers. PPI therapy was soon recognized as being superior for symptom relief and ulcer healing in patients with gastric ulcer disease. Therapy with PPIs resulted in nearly 100% ulcer healing among patients with gastric ulcers responding poorly to H_2RA treatment. Long-term acid-suppression was needed, and H_2RA treatment was usually initiated in patients with a relapse of gastric ulcer disease. Use of prolonged acid suppression with either H_2RA or PPI therapy now seems superseded by effective treatment of *H. pylori* infection. NSAID use is involved in a considerable number of patients with gastric ulcer disease. Termination of NSAID use is one of the most important steps in patient therapy, but PPI treatment seems the best hope for controlling acid secretion and preventing significant ulcer complications when continued NSAID use is essential.

WHEN SHOULD PPI TREATMENT BE ADMINISTERED IN PATIENTS WITH PEPTIC ULCER DISEASE?

1. Effective treatment of *H. pylori* infection in all patients with peptic ulcer disease is universally recommended regardless of whether the patient is undergoing maintenance acid-lowering therapy. Successful treatment of *H. pylori* infection effectively cures peptic ulcer disease. Given the widespread acceptance of PPI triple therapy as effective treatment of *H. pylori* infection in patients, short-term therapy with a PPI seems the best option for symptom control.

2. Effective treatment of *H. pylori* infection is also essential in all patients with complications (e.g., bleeding and perforation) that result from peptic ulcer disease because a dramatic decrease in ulcer recurrence and hence risk of further complications has been demonstrated. Continuation of long-term PPI treatment to prevent ulcer recurrence and successfully treat *H. pylori* infection in older patients, especially those with other serious medical problems, remains somewhat controver-

sial. However, most data strongly suggest that successful treatment of *H. pylori* infection results in few patients having ulcer recurrence and hence complications. There seems little evidence to support the need for long-term maintenance therapy in such patients.

3. PPI treatment is the drug-of-choice in patients with peptic ulcer disease when NSAID therapy needs to be continued. Most studies show that PPI treatment reduces the risk of peptic ulcer disease in patients taking NSAIDs, whilst only one H_2RA (i.e, famotidine in high doses) seems effective. Universal prophylaxis with PPI treatment is probably unjustified. Patients at higher risk of serious gastrointestinal complications should be identified and PPI treatment coprescribed if NSAID use is required. Such patients include those with a documented history of peptic ulcer disease, patients older than 65 years of age, patients who require high doses of NSAID therapy, patients concurrently using NSAIDs and corticosteroids, and patients with significant cardiac or respiratory disease.

ROLE IN *H. PYLORI* ERADICATION

The most convincing evidence to support the causal role of *H. pylori* infection in the pathogenesis of peptic ulcer disease in patients is the dramatic decrease in ulcer recurrence and complication rates following effective treatment of the bacteria. Successful treatment of patients with *H. pylori* infection effectively cures peptic ulcer disease. Further, ulcer healing is accelerated when acid-lowering drugs are used together with effective treatment for *H. pylori* infection. Treatment is recommended for all *H. pylori*-infected patients with peptic ulcer disease and in patients with ulcers who are on long-term acid suppression therapy. Numerous treatment regimens have been studied for the cure of *H. pylori* infection, but the optimum treatment remains to be established. Until recently, the standard approach for *H. pylori* infection in patients was a 14-day course of bismuth-based triple therapy composed of colloidal bismuth, a nitroimidazole (usually metronidazole), and either amoxicillin or tetracycline. Despite cure rates close to 80% in clinical trials, success rates in real world situations have been hampered by side effects, poor patient compliance, and increasing nitroimidazole resistance. Attention soon focused on the use of a PPI in combination with one or more antimicrobial agents because of the proven efficacy of PPI treatment in patients with peptic ulcer disease. Dual therapy comprising a PPI plus amoxicillin for 14 days was a simple alternative to bismuth and proved effective and well tolerated. However, the effective treatment rate varied considerably in a meta-analysis reporting a mean effective treatment rate of only 60% for omeprazole plus amoxicillin and an effective treatment rate of more than 70% when clarithromycin was substituted for amoxicillin. Higher and more consistent rates of effective treatment of *H. pylori* infection in patients have been achieved using a PPI with two or three antibiotics. PPI triple regimens containing clarithromycin appears to be superior to PPI regimens involving amoxicillin. All PPI combination treatments achieve high cure rates and are well tolerated. PPI triple regimens achieve effective 24-hour control of gastric acid secretion and promote rapid symptom resolution and healing of ulcers; the triple regimens provide approximately 90% eradication rates. The combination of a PPI plus two antibiotics for 7 to 10 days has gained acceptance as the current gold standard.

WHEN SHOULD PPI TREATMENT BE ADMINISTERED IN PATIENTS WITH *H. PYLORI* INFECTION?

PPI-based triple therapy is an effective and well-tolerated treatment of patients with peptic ulcer disease. This triple therapy is the treatment regimen of choice in most patients with *H. pylori* infection where cure of the infection is thought necessary. Short-term therapy with a PPI and two antibiotics is better tolerated than bismuth triple therapy, more reliable than dual therapy, simple to administer, and effective in 7 to 10 days.

GASTROESOPHAGEAL REFLUX DISEASE

BACKGROUND

GERD is a common condition in Western societies; approximately 40% of the population experience heartburn at least once a month. Incidence rates of ulcerative esophagitis are considerably lower. GERD results from prolonged exposure of the distal esophagus to the acid contents of the stomach, which is usually related to the incompetence of the lower esophageal sphincter. Heartburn, fluid regurgitation (acid), and dysphagia are major symptoms. These range from mild occasional heartburn and regurgitation without any evidence of macroscopic esophagitis to severe chronic inflammation and ulceration complicated by stricture, bleeding, and anaemia. GERD is divided endoscopically into four stages according to the severity of the mucosal lesion. The clinical spectrum of uncomplicated GERD ranges from reflux symptoms without evidence of esophageal damage (stage 0) to erosive and ulcerative esophagitis (stages II to IV). Severe prolonged exposure of the lower esophageal mucosa to gastric contents may rarely result in histologic change with the development of a columnar-lined esophagus (Barrett's esophagus) that has the greatly increased risk of esophageal adenocarcinoma.

PATHOPHYSIOLOGY

Despite the demonstration of motility disorders, the single most important factor in the pathophysiology of GERD is the abnormal exposure of the esophageal mucosa to gastric acid. The time during a 24-hour period during which the intraesophageal pH level is less than 4 increases progressively from endoscopy negative GERD to the most severe types of esophagitis. Symptoms also correlate with the amount of time the intraesophageal pH level is below 4.

ROLE OF ACID SUPPRESSION

Gastric acid is pivotal to the development of esophageal damage and reflux symptoms in GERD. It therefore follows that suppression of intragastric acid represents the most rational approach to the management of patients with GERD. Meta-analysis predicts effective treatment in more than 90% of patients with ulcerative esophagitis within 8 weeks if the intragastric acidity is maintained above pH level 4 for approximately 21 hours in a 24-hour period. Treatment options for the suppression of gastric acid lie between H_2RA and PPI therapy.

HISTAMINE RECEPTOR ANTAGONISTS

Whilst H_2RA treatment significantly reduces gastric acid secretion through competitive antagonism at the H_2 receptor, stimulation of the gastrin and cholinergic receptors can partially overcome the acid suppression effects of H_2RAs. This limits the drug treatment's ability to control food-stimulated daytime acid secretion, which is a major drawback in most patients with even mild disease since most GERD symptoms occur after meals. Further, tolerance to H_2RA treatment develops early in therapy.

Overall, H_2RA treatment has been less effective in the management of patients with GERD than in patients with peptic ulcer disease. Effective treatment has been recorded in approximately 50% of patients with ulcerative esophagitis when H_2RA treatment is administered in standard doses. Treatment response in patients depends on the grade of the esophageal disease, with the most predictable response being in patients with minor degrees of esophagitis. Fortunately, the vast majority of patients with GERD have minor disease, hence the high efficacy rates of H_2RA treatment. Higher and more frequent doses of H_2RAs are needed to guarantee symptom relief and achieve reasonable endoscopic healing rates in patients with more severe grades of esophagitis.

PROTON PUMP INHIBITORS

In marked contrast to H_2RA treatment, PPI treatment guarantees effective control of gastric acid secretion throughout an entire 24-hour period and no evidence of patient tolerance has been recorded during long-term use. Large clinical trials have confirmed the superiority of PPI treatment over standard dose H_2RAs in regard to both symptom relief and the healing of ulcerative esophagitis in patients with GERD. Although PPI treatment is effective in more than 80% of patients with ulcerative esophagitis after 4 weeks of therapy and more than 90% of patients after 8 weeks of therapy, most H_2RA studies suggest a less than 50% efficacy rate of treatment at 4 weeks and less than 70% at 8 weeks. PPI treatment has also proved effective in patients with GERD who are refractory to prolonged H_2RA treatment. The advantage of PPI treatment over standard dose H_2RA treatment is evident from the most minor to the most severe grades of esophagitis.

LONG-TERM TREATMENT

GERD is not a short-lived problem. Regardless of treatment regimen, most patients experience relapse within a few months of cessation of medical therapy. Long-term medical management is required to control symptoms and manage patients with GERD. Relapse rates in patients with GERD correlate with the degree of esophageal damage. Patients with severe ulcerative esophagitis invariably relapse within 6 months of discontinuing acute therapy with a PPI. The relapse rate of mild esophagitis after H$_2$RA treatment is less predictable and less frequent. Remission can be maintained in the majority of patients by long-term acid suppression. Nearly all patients undergoing long-term PPI treatment remain symptom-free. However, it still would seem reasonable to reserve long-term PPI treatment for those patients in whom H$_2$RA treatment fails to achieve a reasonable symptomatic response because the majority of patients with GERD have mild esophagitis that is reasonably managed with long-term H$_2$RA treatment. Yet PPI treatment is increasingly becoming recognized as first line therapy for the short- and long-term management of patients with GERD. It provides more efficient and more predictable treatment and symptom resolution across all grades of esophagitis, and PPI treatment is more effective in managing patients in remission. These benefits may confer greater cost-effectiveness for PPI treatment by permitting shorter treatment periods for acute therapy, having fewer treatment failures, preventing more disease recurrence, and therefore reducing the need for excessive medical consultation and investigation. The superior clinical efficacy of PPI treatment is clearly evidenced in the greater degree and duration of acid suppression achieved in patients, particularly after meals.

No evidence exists indicating *H. pylori* infection may cause GERD. Effective treatment of coexistent *H. pylori* infection is therefore unlikely to provide additional therapeutic benefit in patients with GERD. Theoretically, long-term powerful gastric acid suppression in *H. pylori*-infected patients with chronic gastritis may induce harmful mucosal changes and place the patient at risk for developing gastric cancer. Hence, some experts suggest effective treatment of *H. pylori* infection is an important initial step in patients with ulcerative reflux disease who require long-term PPI therapy. More long-term data are required.

Surgical procedures on the lower esophagus, particularly laparoscopic fundoplication, remains another option and should be considered in all patients younger than 50 years of age with ulcerative GERD requiring long-term acid suppression with PPI treatment.

COMPLICATIONS

1. Most complications in patients with GERD arise from the ulcerated inflamed esophageal mucosa. Patient treatment with long-term antisecretory therapy (usually PPI) may prevent complications such as esophageal stricture. PPI treatment is more effective than H_2RA treatment in relieving dysphagia and reducing the need for repeat dilatation in patients with an esophageal stricture complicating GERD.

WHEN SHOULD PPI TREATMENT BE ADMINISTERED IN PATIENTS WITH GASTROESOPHAGEAL REFLUX DISEASE?

1. Most patients with GERD have mild disease with minor symptoms and respond well to H_2RA treatment.

2. Patients with ulcerative reflux disease usually require more powerful acid suppression, and studies suggest that PPI treatment is the current drug of choice for first line and maintenance therapy in such patients.

ZOLLINGER-ELLISON SYNDROME

Zollinger-Ellison Syndrome (ZE) is an uncommon disease usually located in the pancreas and is related to gastrin cell tumors. ZE is characterized by severe recurrent peptic ulcer disease, high levels of gastric acid secretion, and high circulating levels of gastrin. Therapy for patients with ZE includes treatment of the often malignant neoplasm and control of gastric acid hyper-secretion. Total gastrectomy was the treatment of choice to eliminate acid secretion in patients until the development of acid-lowering medication. H_2RA treatment allows control of intractable peptic ulcer disease. Long-term maintenance therapy combined with tumor removal when possible became the favored approach. PPI treatment quickly replaced H_2RA treatment because of its powerful acid suppression. PPI treatment achieves symptom control and provides effective treatment of ulcers in the majority of patients. Although PPI doses are higher for effective acid inhibition in patients with ZE than in patients with simple peptic ulcer disease, a single daily dose is initially capable of inhibiting gastric acid secretion in 80% of patients with ZE. The other 20% of patients require twice daily dosing. Patient tolerance to PPI treatment is observed less frequently than with H_2RA treatment. Few patients with gastrinoma undergoing PPI treatment require dose changes each year. Early tumor recognition and excision are of primary importance in patient management because PPI treatment successfully controls gastric acid secretion and the current major cause of mortality in patients with ZE is widespread metastatic disease.

WHEN SHOULD PPI TREATMENT BE ADMINISTERED IN PATIENTS WITH ZOLLINGER-ELLISON SYNDROME?

PPI treatment has replaced H_2RA treatment in the management of patients with ZE because of its marked potency, prolonged duration of action, and safety profile. PPI treatment has led to a significant decrease in mortality rates related to complications of acid-peptic disease, particularly bleeding and perforation.

FUNCTIONAL DYSPEPSIA

Dyspepsia is one of the most frequently recorded health problems in Western communities. Epidemiologic studies have reported annual prevalence rates at approximately 25% when dyspepsia is defined as upper abdominal symptoms and heartburn is excluded. Most patients with dyspepsia do not seek medical attention. Functional (i.e., non-ulcer) dyspepsia is a heterogeneous disorder characterized by recurrent or chronic upper abdominal discomfort or pain that is not the result of an organic disorder such as peptic ulcer disease, gastric cancer, gallstones, GERD, or chronic pancreatitis. Disorders of gastrointestinal function such as delayed gastric emptying are found in some patients, but the relationship of this finding to symptoms remains poorly understood.

The current rationale for drug treatment is based on altering pathophysiologic mechanisms that are believed to be associated with symptom development. Despite many studies showing placebo response rates approach 60%, prokinetic agents such as cisapride, acid-suppressing agents, and bismuth-containing compounds are more effective than placebos in reducing symptoms. Antacids are widely used, but no control study has been able to demonstrate a significant benefit over placebos. First line treatment includes the exclusion of organic disease, reassurance and explanation of their symptoms, and avoidance of precipitating factors. Identifying optimal medication for a patient continues to be a trial and error process. Many patients with functional dyspepsia have symptoms that may be reflective of acid-related disorder (i.e., ulcer-like dyspepsia). Some patients with functional dyspepsia have histologically documented inflammation of the gastric and duodenal mucosa. Such inflammation may be controlled if acid secretion is reduced temporally or permanently. Thus, drugs aimed towards the suppression of acid secretion have been frequently administered.

Analysis suggests there is a therapeutic advantage to using H_2RA treatment compared with placebo. Patients with typical ulcer-like symptoms or coexistent symptomatic GERD are most likely to respond. Powerful acid suppression could be valuable in patients with severe symptoms of functional dyspepsia. However, functional dyspepsia is a benign disorder, and the use of a PPI in such a disease must remain questionable until the efficacy of such drugs has been established and their long-term safety guaranteed. Despite this caveat, a trial of a PPI may be justified if it is administered under close medical supervision to a limited number of patients with troublesome symptoms who do not respond to conventional acid suppression (usually H_2RA treatment). The benefits of effective treatment of *H. pylori* infection on dyspeptic symptoms is far from established. Bismuth-containing agents may have beneficial effects on patients with dyspepsia, but this seems independent of the agents' role in effective treatment of *H. pylori* infection.

WHEN SHOULD PPI TREATMENT BE ADMINISTERED IN PATIENTS WITH FUNCTIONAL DYSPEPSIA?

The optimal management of functional dyspepsia should take into account the intensity and duration of patient symptoms and the impact of symptoms on the patient's quality of life. The challenge is to select patients who will benefit from a particular medication regimen and to determine the duration of treatment. Empiric treatment will dominate clinical practice until clinicians better understand the mechanisms causing functional dyspepsia. PPI treatment may have an occasional role in such empiric therapy.

CONCLUSION

The treatment of acid-related disorders such as peptic ulcer disease and GERD in patients has been revolutionized during the previous 20 years. H_2RA treatment has proved safe, effective, and convenient for the relief of symptoms and is effective treatment in the majority of patients with peptic ulcer disease.

However, H_2RA treatment is relatively ineffective in patients with ulcerative reflux disease. A new class of drug, the PPI, was introduced in the late 1980s. These drugs suppress gastric acid secretion by inhibiting H^+,K^+-ATPase, which is the gastric proton pump, located in the secretory membrane of the parietal cell. PPIs produce profound inhibition of acid secretion because they block the final step in the production of gastric acid, and the covalent nature of their binding to the pump leads to a long duration of action. The resultant pharmacology leads to more efficient treatment and symptom relief in patients with peptic ulcer disease compared to H_2RA treatment and provides effective symptom relief and treatment in patients with GERD. The medical management of patients with ZE has been transformed by PPI treatment, which provides rapid relief of symptoms, effective treatment of ulcers, and prevention of the devastating complications of bleeding and perforation. The pivotal role of *H. pylori* infection in patients with peptic ulcer disease has been established. PPI treatment with two or three antibiotics in a short-term therapeutic regimen seems well established, and such regimens are becoming the gold standard for effectively treating patients with *H. pylori* infection. PPI treatment is the therapy of choice in most patients with ulceration that results from acid-related disorders.

SUGGESTED READINGS

Bardhan KD. Triple therapy as a cure for *Helicobacter pylori* infection. Eur J Gastroenterol Hepatol 1996;8(Suppl 1):S27–S30 (This article is a comprehensive review of triple therapy including PPI triple as therapy of *H. Pylori* infection.)

Bell NJV, Burget D, Howden CW, et al. Appropriate acid suppression for the management of gastroesophageal reflux disease. Digestion 1992;51:59–67. (This is an important meta-analysis that documents appropriate levels of acid suppression required for management of GERD.)

Black JW, Duncan WAM, Durant CJ, et al. Definitions and antagonism of histamine H_2 receptors. Nature 1972;236:385–390. (This landmark article established the importance of Histamine H_2 receptors in acid secretion and acknowledged the possibility of the important role of Histamine H_2 receptor antagonists in acid secretion.)

Brunner G, Creutzfeldt W. Omeprazole in the long-term management of patients with acid-related resistant to ranitidine. Scand J Gastroenterol 1989;166:101–105. (This article is shows the efficacy of the first PPI omeprazole in managing patients with esophagitis and peptic ulcers that are resistant to an H$_2$RA, ranitidine.)

Sachs G. The gastric H, K ATPase, regulation and structure/function of the acid pump of the stomach. In: Johnson LR, ed. Physiology of the Gastrointestinal Tract. Philadelphia: Raven Press, 1994:1119. (This is a classic review of the gastric acid proton pump.)

Sachs G, Shin JM, Bejancon M, Prinz C. The continuing development of gastric acid pump inhibitors. Aliment Pharmacol Ther 1993;7(Suppl 1):4–12. (This is an excellent review of the development and clinical application of PPIs.)

Chapter Three

IRRITABLE BOWEL SYNDROME: PRESENT AND FUTURE APPROACHES TO TREATMENT

Tony Lembo, MD, Lin Chang, MD, and
Emeran A. Mayer, MD

INTRODUCTION

Irritable bowel syndrome (IBS) is a chronic disorder of unknown etiology characterized by exacerbations of abdominal pain and discomfort and alterations in bowel movements. IBS affects approximately 22% of the United States population, and patients with this disorder account for approximately 28% of patients seen by gastroenterologists. Diagnostic criteria has been recently established, and existing diagnostic and therapeutic guidelines are empirical and not supported by well-controlled clinical trials. This chapter reviews evolving concepts on the etiology of IBS, the diagnostic criteria for diagnosing IBS in patients, and disease management of patients with IBS.

EPIDEMIOLOGY

Based on random samples, between 9% and 22% of the United States and western European population report symptoms consistent with IBS. The prevalence is similar in Japan, China, South America, and India. Women have higher incidence rates of IBS than men. The elderly appear to be less prone to IBS than the general population. Approximately 25% of patients report onset of symptoms within the previous year. The prevalence of IBS is similar in Caucasian and African American patients, although it may be lower in Hispanic patients.

The presence, location, and character of gastrointestinal (GI) symptoms in patients with IBS are not constant over time. A longitudinal study using questionnaires one year and six months after initial contact showed 38% of patients with IBS had resolution of their symptoms and 9% of those surveyed who had not initially reported IBS symptoms had symptoms consistent with IBS. Another study using questionnaires one year after initial contact revealed 22% of patients whose symptoms were initially classified as characteristic of IBS experienced symptoms consistent with functional dyspepsia and 16% of patients whose symptoms were originally classified as characteristic of functional dyspepsia experienced symptoms associated with IBS. These findings suggest that IBS and at least a subset of functional dyspepsia are related disorders that can manifest in the same patient at different times or can coexist in approximately 90% of patients.

Although symptoms of IBS are common in the general population, only 9% of people with IBS symptoms seek medical care. Factors that predict if individuals with IBS seek medical treatment include severity of abdominal pain, psychological disturbances, stressful or traumatic life events, and cultural factors. For example, men predominate in IBS clinics in India. Although only a small percentage of people seek medical care, the symptoms of IBS result in more than 3.5 million physician visits and more than 2.2 million prescriptions per year in the United States.

The exact cost of IBS to the economy is unknown but probably is substantial. Subjects in Olmsted County, MN, who reported symptoms consistent with IBS on postal questionnaires incurred 1.6 times more medical charges than subjects without IBS symptoms during the year prior to the survey. Patients with IBS undergo more surgical and other procedures, which are frequently unnecessary (e.g., appendectomies, cholecystectomies, and hysterectomies), than patients with other GI disorders. In a United Stated survey, subjects who had symptoms consistent with IBS missed nearly three times as many work days in the year prior to the survey as did subjects who did not report IBS symptoms. Thus, the costs to society from direct medical expenditures and from loss of patient productivity are substantial.

ETIOLOGY

The etiology of IBS remains poorly understood. The most pertinent question regarding IBS is what factors differentiate the individuals who experience occasional IBS-like symptomology but consider themselves healthy from the patients who experience chronic IBS symptomology and require medical treatment. Although the answer to this question is unknown, clinical evidence strongly suggests genetic factors. Although IBS symptoms are experienced by a high percentage of the healthy population, a medical syndrome will develop only in a subset of the population that has other risk factors that make such a transition likely.

Recent data suggest genetic predisposition may contribute to the development of IBS in some patients. Symptoms consistent with IBS are more common in first-degree relatives but not spouses of subjects with IBS. Additionally, in an Australian study of twins, a proportion of the incidence of IBS in both twins was felt to be the result of genetic rather than environmental factors.

Early life events are important in the expression of IBS symptoms later in life. Patients with IBS differ from nonpatients (those who have not sought medical care for IBS) in the amount of attention they received for common physical ailments during their youth. The frequency of absenteeism from school and visits to the pediatrician is also higher in patients with IBS than non-patients. This conditioning in early life may result in the development of illness behavior or an over-reporting of physical ailments in an attempt to receive attention and affection. Other significant early life events such as major traumatic events (e.g., physical or sexual abuse) or major losses (e.g., the loss of a parent) during childhood are present more frequently in patients with IBS than healthy control patients. Taken together, these data suggest that early life events are important in the expression of IBS symptomology and possibly the pathogenesis of IBS later in life.

Stressful events are often reported by patients to precede the onset or exacerbation of IBS symptoms. In a questionnaire study of 135 patients with IBS and 654 control subjects, 73% of patients with IBS and 54% of control subjects reported stress altered their stool pattern and 84% of patients with IBS and 68% of control subjects reported stress led to abdominal pain. Stress also correlates with the frequency of bowel symptoms (such as abdominal pain and cramps and altered stool patterns) and the number of disability days and physician visits. In addition to daily stressors, a history of severe emotional trauma such as physical and sexual abuse, especially when incurred during childhood, is associated with increased risk of developing IBS. In a study at the University of North Carolina, 53% of women with IBS had a history of abuse in comparison to 37% of women with structural GI diagnoses. Not surprisingly, patients who experienced life-threatening events, which resulted in post-traumatic stress disorder, also have a high incidence of IBS.

Comorbid psychiatric diagnoses (the most common being depression and generalized anxiety disorder) are present in approximately 42 to 61% of patients with IBS referred to a tertiary referral center. IBS non-patients, on the other hand, have psychological characteristics similar to the general population. Many questions remain regarding this high degree of comorbidity, including: (1) is this high degree of comorbidity a consequence of having a chronic disease that severely impacts (such as abdominal pain and cramps and altered stool patterns) quality of life, (2) is the comorbidity a random co-occurrence of common disorders, and (3) do the central nervous system alterations underlying affective disorders and changes in visceral sensory and autonomic regulation affect similar neurophysiologic mechanisms. Many patients with IBS also have ineffective coping skills for symptom management and dealing with stress in general.

IBS symptoms occur in approximately 33% of patients after acute GI infection and often persist for years following complete resolution of infection. Psychometric scores for anxiety, depression, somatization, and neurotic traits are higher at the time of infection in those patients who develop IBS symptoms than those patients who return to normal bowel function. In psychologically susceptible patients, enteric infections and presumably other causes of mucosal irritation can precipitate IBS symptoms that may persist after the infection or inflammation has resolved.

Food intolerance is commonly reported by patients with IBS. However, a causal relationship between intake of certain foods and IBS symptoms has not been established. Carbohydrate intolerance is unlikely to play a significant role in symptom generation in most patients with IBS; the prevalence of carbohydrate malabsorption is similar in patients with IBS to that in asymptomatic control subjects, and treating patients with IBS with lactase has not been shown to affect IBS symptoms. Likewise, exclusionary diets in comparison to placebo have not been effective in improving IBS symptoms in most patients. IBS symptoms do not improve in patients with positive skin test responses to particular foods after the patients eliminate those foods from their diet. Thus, although patients often report specific food intolerances, it is more likely that patients have developed a conditioned response to food intake, which may develop as a result of non-specific exacerbation of abdominal symptoms by switching the GI tract from a fasting to a fed pattern, and this is not a true hypersensitivity to a specific food component.

Several abnormal motor patterns have been reported in patients with IBS. These patterns are nonspecific and rarely correlate with symptoms, which suggests these responses are a secondary phenomena rather than a primary motility disorder. Several studies have shown hypermotility of the rectosigmoid colon in response to eating or stressful interviews, which may explain why many patients with IBS experience typical IBS symptoms after meals or develop exacerbation of symptoms during stressful life events.

The lack of correlation between symptoms and abnormal intestinal motility has resulted in a refocusing of research efforts into identifying alterations in visceral sensations as a cause of IBS symptoms. Several studies have reported that IBS patients report discomfort and pain at lower distention intensities when balloons are inflated throughout the gastrointestinal tract. These findings do not appear to be secondary to alterations in intestinal tone or compliance, nor do they correlate with measures of psychoneuroticism. IBS patients appear to be more vigilant towards unpleasant visceral sensations, show alterations in viscerosomatic referral, and demonstrate a unique hyperalgesic response to repetitive distention of the sigmoid colon. Consistent with the reported alterations in the perception of visceral afferent information, specific alterations in regional brain activity have recently been reported in patients with IBS. In contrast to other physiologic mechanisms proposed to explain symptom generation in IBS patients, alterations in processing of viscerosensory information has been the most reproducible marker of this disorder.

PATHOPHYSIOLOGY

Although the pathophysiology of IBS is not completely understood, a multicomponent model of IBS, which is similar to other chronic illness and involves physiologic, affective, cognitive, and behavioral factors, can be formulated. The importance of each factor in the generation of IBS symptoms may vary greatly between person to person. Physiologic factors implicated in the generation of IBS symptoms include hypersensitivity of the GI tract to normal events; autonomic dysfunction including altered intestinal motility response to stress, anger, and food intake; changes in fluid and electrolyte processing by the bowel; and alterations in sleep. However, alterations in these physiologic parameters are generally only found in subsets of patients and, in the case of intestinal dysmotility, frequently do not correlate with symptoms. Approximately 60% of patients with IBS report behavioral factors, such as stressful life events, to be associated with the onset or exacerbation of their symptoms. Patient characteristics such as inappropriate coping mechanisms and inaccurate theories on disease, nutrition, and medications are common in patients with IBS, and these cognitive factors influence patients in seeking professional treatment and improving clinical outcomes. Affective disorders are present in a large percentage of patients with IBS seeking treatment and are primarily manifested in the form of anxiety, panic disorder, and depression. Patients with IBS may also be hypervigilant to visceral stimuli.

CLINICAL FEATURES

IBS has been defined as recurrent GI symptoms not explained by structural or biochemical abnormalities that are related to the intestines and associated with symptoms of pain or discomfort as well as disturbed defecation, feelings of being bloated, and abdominal distention. Manning et al were the first to report six symptoms which occurred more commonly in patients with IBS than in patients with other GI illnesses; these have since become known as the Manning Criteria. Each of these symptoms, however, was present in at least 20% of the control group, which consisted of patients with organic GI illnesses. Subsequent studies have shown that the sensitivity and specificity of the Manning Criteria are 58% and 74%, respectively, in differentiating IBS from organic disease. More recently an international report on functional bowel disorders developed a consensus definition and criteria for IBS, which is known as the "Rome" criteria. The accuracy of the international criteria has yet to be reported, but this clinical definition of IBS is probably the safest and most reasonable for diagnosing IBS.

IBS patients tend to present with multiple GI and non-GI symptoms. Some GI symptoms commonly reported include dyspepsia, nausea and vomiting, heartburn, and globus sensation. Some non-GI symptoms frequently reported include increased urinary frequency and urgency especially in women with IBS, sexual impairment, fibromyalgia and other rheumatologic symptoms, lower back pain, headaches, and nonspecific fatigue (e.g., chronic fatigue syndrome). Although patients with IBS tend to report multiple non-GI symptoms, they do not have a lower tolerance to pain; patients with IBS are able to tolerate cold water hand immersion and heat stimulation as well as healthy patients.

DIAGNOSIS

Physical findings and diagnostic tests lack sufficient specificity in diagnosing IBS in patients. The diagnosis of IBS is based on symptom criteria and the exclusion of organic disease. A detailed history using established symptom criteria often can exclude the majority of organic diseases that could cause symptoms consistent with IBS. A careful history and physical examination should include documentation of features suggestive of organic disease such as bleeding, weight loss, and anemia.

The diagnostic evaluation administered to rule out organic disease in patients with symptoms compatible with IBS is guided by patient's symptomology and history. For example, patients older than 50 years of age with new-onset, changing, or severe symptoms should undergo a more detailed evaluation, which includes a colonoscopy; patients with mild or moderate symptoms who are younger than 50 years of age and do not have symptoms of organic disease should undergo a limited diagnostic evaluation. Initial diagnostic evaluation of patients with diarrhea-predominant IBS should include stool evaluation for ova and parasites if the patients have new-onset symptoms, have recently traveled, or are immunocompromised. The initial evaluation of patients with long-standing diarrhea-predominant IBS should include the following testing: stool guaiac, complete blood count, thyroid function, and stool for white cell count. Patients with constipation-predominant IBS do not need an evaluation for GI infections. The initial evaluation of these patients should include the following: paradoxic pelvic floor contraction if decreased frequency of bowel movements is present and flexible sigmoidoscopy if rectal fullness is present or a colonic transit study to rule out colonic inertia.

Behavioral and psychological assessment is essential for cost-effective evaluation of patients with IBS. Appropriate patient assessment is obtained by taking a detailed patient history, being familiar with the most common psychological symptoms and life stressors, and administering simple questionnaires (SCL-90) or using a multidisciplinary approach that involves a mental health professional. The latter approach should probably be reserved for tertiary referral centers evaluating a patient population with the highest prevalence and greatest severity of behavioral and psychological disturbances.

TREATMENT

The efficacy of current pharmacologic and psychological therapies remains in question. An extensive review of randomized, double-blind, placebo-controlled drug trials performed between 1966 and 1988 by Klein found that none of the studies provided statistical evidence suggesting any of the medications were beneficial in treating IBS symptoms. Most studies were flawed because of short treatment periods (approximately 50% were less than 4 weeks in duration), poor operational definition of IBS, crossover design (which is flawed because of the carry-over effect), and a short or no follow-up period. A recent critical review of psychotherapies for IBS by Talley also found no therapy is better than placebo and most of the studies are flawed. Despite the lack of reliable controlled outcome data, a general consensus exists that pharmacologic and behavioral approaches can improve specific symptoms such as abdominal pain, diarrhea, and constipation and alleviate anxiety and depression.

FIBER

Dietary fiber adds nondigestable bulk to stool by retaining water because of its hydrophilic properties and by serving as a substrate for microbial growth in the colon. Fiber limits stool dehydration and normalizes stool consistency by absorbing water. Colonic transit time in normal and constipated patients is reduced by dietary fiber at doses ranging from approximately 12 to 20 g. Commonly used fiber supplements for IBS symptoms include psyllium (Metamucil, Konsyl, FibroCon), methylcellulose (Citrocel), and polycarbophil (Fiberall, Fibercon). Patients should be warned that bloating and abdominal distention may occur, especially at the beginning of therapy, and will usually disappear spontaneously after several weeks or by diminishing the fiber dose. A prudent approach is to start a patient on a minimal twice daily dosage (e.g., a teaspoon two times a day) and gradually increase the dose of fiber to the maximally tolerated amount over several weeks. Despite the widespread use of fiber, particularly for constipation-predominant IBS, multiple controlled studies have failed to show the overall value of fiber in the treatment of IBS symptoms.

ANTIDIARRHEAL AGENTS

Antidiarrheal agents such as synthetic opioids (e.g., diphenoxylate [Lomotil], loperamide [Imodium]) are effective in reducing the frequency of diarrhea in patients with IBS. Synthetic opioids reduce gut motility and secretion, which allows for greater fluid resorption and improved stool consistency. Several clinical trials have demonstrated opioid's ability to improve stool frequency and consistency and alleviate fecal urgency associated with IBS.

SMOOTH MUSCLE RELAXANTS

Smooth muscle relaxants or antispasmodics are thought to relieve abdominal symptoms by inhibiting intestinal smooth muscle contractions and thereby decreasing colonic motor activity. Agents included in this class are anticholinergics and calcium channel blockers. A recent meta-analysis by Poynard et al of 26 randomized controlled trials with eight different drugs concluded that smooth muscle relaxants were better than placebo for global assessment (62% versus 35%) and abdominal pain (64% versus 45%). No improvement was detected in patients with constipation or abdominal distention. When the eight drugs were analyzed separately, the following three drugs had efficacy in comparison to placebo: cimetropium bromide (Alginor, Italy), dicyclomine bromide (Bentyl), which is a antimuscarinic compound, and octylonium (Spasmomen, Spain), which is a quaternary ammonium derivative with calcium-antagonist properties. These compounds may work in a subset of patients in whom enhanced, more frequent, or prolonged intestinal motor activity contributes to symptoms. Alternatively, the CNS effect of these compounds, which includes sedation, may also play a role in symptom relief.

PROKINETIC AGENTS

Available prokinetic agents have had a limited role in treating patients with constipation-predominant IBS. Cisapride, which is a serotonin receptor agonist [$5HT_3$] and antagonist [$5HT_4$])

and increases acetylcholine release from the myenteric plexus, has been shown to increase lower esophageal sphincter pressure and amplitude of esophageal contractions, accelerate gastric emptying of solids and liquids, and increase small bowel motor activity. Cisapride also accelerates colonic transit, but this effect may be greater in right colon than left.

Cisapride treatment in patients with IBS has been studied in two placebo-controlled studies. Van Outryve et al conducted a randomized, double-blind, placebo-controlled study in 69 patients with constipation-predominant IBS. The dose of cisapride ranged from 2.5 to 10 mg and was administered orally three times a day during a 12-week study duration. Stool frequency and number of days with normal stools increased for cisapride and placebo groups by week four and continued to improve in the cisapride group and remained unchanged in the placebo group during weeks eight to 12. Abdominal pain and abdominal distention decreased in both groups by week four, but the alleviation of symptoms was greater in the cisapride group than placebo group by week 12. The overall rating for response to treatment at week 12 was good or excellent in 71% in the cisapride group versus 39% in the placebo group. The agent was well tolerated. Another study by Hurlimann et al reported a decrease in bloating in patients with bloating-predominant IBS who were treated with 10 mg of cisapride administered orally three times a day for 4 weeks compared to placebo ($p < 0.05$).

Researchers have not determined the exact mechanism by which cisapride may improve the symptoms of constipation. The mechanism may include increasing coordination of colonic peristaltic activity and reducing the sensory threshold for urge to defecate. Additional well-designed trials are needed to determine the drug's long-term efficacy and to determine if cisapride is beneficial for all patients with chronic constipation or only for specific subgroups. At present, the recommended dose of cisapride for treatment of patients with functional constipation is 5 to 10 mg administered orally three times a day 15 to 30 minutes before meals. Other prokinetic agents such as metoclopramide, domperidone, and erythromycin have no significant efficacy as treatment of IBS symptoms in patients.

ANTIDEPRESSANTS AND ANXIOLYTICS

Antidepressants have been used as treatment for patients with chronic pain because of their analgesic action and antidepressant effect. An uncontrolled retrospective review by Clouse et al reviewed the efficacy of antidepressants on overall improvement in 138 patients with IBS. The antidepressant agents that were reviewed are listed in descending order of frequency: amitriptyline (10 to 125 mg/d), doxepin (10 to 100 mg/d), amoxapine (25 to 200 mg/d), alprazolam (0.25 to 2.25 mg/d), thioridazine (10 to 40 mg/d), trazodone (50 to 150 mg/d), protriptyline (5 to 15 mg/d), and imipramine (20 to 25 mg/d). Global improvement occurred in 89% of patients, and remission of symptoms occurred in 61%. Despite the limitations of the study, several observations were made: (1) the response rate was greatest for patients with pain-predominant IBS (81%) as compared to patients with diarrhea-predominant IBS (60%) and constipation-predominant IBS (51%); (2) improvement and remission occurred with lower dose treatment regimens of antidepressants (50 mg/day of several of the tricyclic antidepressants); and (3) psychiatric features did not influence clinical response. Despite the use of low doses, side effects including sedation and anticholinergic effects occurred in 30% of patients, and 58% of those patients required change to alternative antidepressant treatment regimens. Similar to what was recorded for patients with chronic somatic pain conditions, psychiatric comorbidity did not influence clinical response rates. The mechanism of action of antidepressants given in non-psychiatric doses is unknown, but it likely involves effects on supraspinal structures.

Treatment with full antidepressant doses of selective serotonin reuptake inhibitors is only indicated in patients with established comorbid diagnoses of depression or anxiety disorder. No studies have been published on the possible effects of these compounds in patients with IBS who do not have a psychiatric diagnosis. Several new visceral analgesics are currently in various stages of clinical development.

VISCERAL ANALGESICS

The long-acting somatostatin analogue, octreotide, is useful in treating patients with visceral and somatic chronic pain syndromes. Octreotide was recently studied for its effect on afferent rectal sensation in healthy patients and patients with IBS. Subcutaneous injections of octreotide (approximately 100 mg) in normal patients increased pressure and volume thresholds of non-noxious and noxious sensations during slow ramp distention (20 to 100 ml/min) of the rectum but not rapid ramp (400 ml/min) or phasic distention. These findings and octreotide's lack of effect on the rectoanal inhibitory reflex and receptive relaxation suggest that octreotide alters conscious perception of rectal sensations through inhibition of extrinsic afferent neurons projecting from the mucosa. In patients with diarrhea-predominant IBS, octreotide increases discomfort volume thresholds to ramp distention in comparison to placebo and shifts the pressure-volume curve to the right, which suggests octreotide increases compliance and thereby increases the volume necessary to trigger a sensation. No direct effect on visceral afferent thresholds by octreotide was demonstrated in this study.

Fedotozine, a peripheral κ opioid receptor antagonist, was recently tested in a double-blind, randomized, placebo-controlled multicenter trial. In the trial, 277 patients were randomized to receive either oral fedotozine (30 mg three times a day) or placebo for 6 weeks. Greater improvement of abdominal pain occurred with fedotozine compared to placebo. No difference was noted with respect to transit disorders, bloating, adverse events, and number of withdrawals.

Serotonin ($5HT_3$)-receptor antagonists have been identified in the central nervous system and on postganglionic autonomic, enteric, and sensory neurons. $5HT_3$-receptor antagonists have antiemetic and possibly anxiolytic and analgesic effects. The effect of $5HT_3$-receptor antagonists on rectal sensitivity and intestinal contractility has been studied in patients with IBS. Granisetron, a $5HT_3$-receptor antagonist, decreased rectal sensitivity, which was measured by serial rectal balloon inflations, with increasing volumes in a dose-dependent manner. The rectal postprandial motility index was reduced in a dose-dependent manner with granisetron. There was no effect on anal canal pressures, rectal compliance, and distention-induced motor activity. However, ondansetron, another $5HT_3$-receptor antagonist, had no effect on rectal sensitivity, rectal tone, colonic tone, and the fasting colonic motility index in patients with diarrhea-predominant IBS or healthy subjects. Rectal sensitivity was measured during isobaric ramp-step distentions using a barostat system. The lack of effect of ondansetron was thought to be the result of the 0.15 mg/kg dose, which was administered intravenously and used for its antiemetic activity.

A randomized, double-blind, placebo-controlled crossover trial assessed oral ondansetron's effect on bowel symptoms and intestinal transit in patients with diarrhea-predominant IBS. After treatment with ondansetron, a significant improvement occurred in stool consistency but not in stool frequency, stool weight, and abdominal pain. Ondansetron had a tendency to slow colonic transit but this was not statistically significant. Small intestinal transit was unchanged by this drug. The authors suggest these findings reflect an alteration in the visceral perception of unsatisfactory defecation by ondansetron and not an alteration in intestinal transit. Perhaps, future larger studies using these compounds with standardized validated methods of measuring visceral sensation and bowel symptoms will determine if these agents are efficacious in the treatment of patients with IBS and also the mechanism by which these agents may act.

PSYCHOLOGICAL AND BEHAVIORAL TREATMENT

Psychological treatments being used to treat patients with IBS include: relaxation therapy, biofeedback therapy, hypnosis, psychotherapy (dynamic, cognitive, and cognitive-behavioral therapy), and combination treatment with two or more of the above mentioned treatment options. It is not yet known if one psychological treatment is superior to another or which patients are likely to benefit from which regimens. Therefore, the choice of treatment depends on patient preference, cost, and availability.

Relaxation therapy has been shown to improve symptoms in patients with IBS in randomized controlled trials. The effects of relaxation techniques last for up to four years.

Biofeedback was initially used to treat patients with IBS by modifying colonic motility either by using a stethoscope to alter bowel sounds or by using a rectal balloon to reduce contractile activity. Further studies proved these methods to be ineffective. Biofeedback combined with muscle relaxation training and stress reduction have been reported to be helpful in reducing bowel symptoms such as rectal urgency and abdominal discomfort in patients with IBS, and sustained improvement rates were recorded in up to 50% of patients at four years follow-up. However, no difference between the active treatment group and the placebo group was found when these techniques were studied in placebo-controlled studies. Another study found that these behavioral techniques were similar to medications in treating IBS symptoms.

Hypnosis has been shown to improve IBS symptoms in several studies. For example, hypnosis improved symptoms in approximately 85% of patients in a study with more than 200 patients with IBS. Hypnosis is most effective in patients without associated psychopathology.

Patients can identify stressors and cognitions that may increase physical distress while undergoing cognitive-behavioral therapy. Once identified, coping strategies are developed, thought processes are restructured, and actions are modified to reduce health care utilization. Cognitive-behavioral therapy alone and in combination with other therapies has been shown to improve symptoms in patients with IBS. For example, symptoms improved in almost 65% of patients with IBS when cognitive-behavioral therapy was combined with education and relaxation therapy.

Psychodynamic therapy involves exploring the patient's physical symptoms in great depth, identifying any possible associations between the patient's physical symptoms and their psychological state, and trying to change any such links. In a controlled study by Guthrie et al, 6 sessions of brief psychodynamic therapy (relaxation being a prominent component) combined with medical therapy was compared with medical therapy alone in 102 patients with IBS. The group receiving psychotherapy showed more improvement in diarrhea symptoms, lessening of abdominal pain, alleviation in depression and anxiety, and a decrease in the number of patient visits. Thus, psychotherapy should be a treatment option in patients with moderate to severe IBS symptoms or with psychosocial comorbidities.

CONCLUSION

Treating the symptoms of IBS is challenging because the pathophysiologic mechanisms involved in symptom generation and expression are not well understood. The establishment of a effective patient-physician relationship is essential for the successful treatment of patients with IBS. Once a strong relationship has been formed, a physician can provide the reassurance necessary to alleviate any fears a patient may have about organic disease and can individualize patient treatment regimens. Further research on functional bowel disorders will undoubtedly result in greater therapeutic options in the near future.

SUGGESTED READINGS

Agreus L, Svaerdsudd K, Nyren O, et al. Irritable bowel syndrome and dyspepsia in the general population: overlap and lack of stability over time. Gastroenterology 1995;109:671–680. (At 1-year follow-up, 22% of patients who initially had symptoms of IBS on a questionnaire survey had symptoms consistent with functional dyspepsia, while 16% of patients who were initially classified as functional dyspepsia on initial screening, experienced symptoms associated with IBS at 1-year follow-up. This study suggests that functional gastrointestinal symptoms vary over time and that symptoms frequently change from the upper gastrointestinal tract to the lower tract and vice versa.)

Drossman DA, McKee DC, Sandler RS, et al. Psychosocial factors in the irritable bowel syndrome. A multivariate study of patients and nonpatients with irritable bowel syndrome. Gastroenterology 1988;95:701–708. (Subjects with IBS who had sought medical care for their symptoms showed significantly greater illness behavior and abnormal personality patterns than subjects with IBS who had not sought medical care for their symptoms [IBS non-patients]. IBS non-patients had similar psychological 'score' as did normals, which suggests that psychological factors are associated with whether the patient seeks medical care for their symptoms rather than with the disorder itself.)

Drossman DA, Sandler RS, McKee DC. Bowel patterns among subjects not seeking health care. Gastroenterology 1982;83:529–534. (Using a bowel symptom questionnaire, approximately 17% of subjects not seeking medical care for gastrointestinal symptoms reported bowel dysfunction. Subjects reporting bowel dysfunction were predominantly female and stress influenced their bowel function.)

Gwee KA, Graham JC, McKendrick MW, et al. Psychometric scores and persistence of irritable bowel after infectious diarrhea. Lancet 1996;347:150–153. (Patients who were hospitalized with infectious diarrhea who had IBS symptoms 6 months after discharge had higher initial psychometric scores for anxiety, depression, somatization, and neurotic trait than did patients whose bowel habits returned to normal. This suggests that patients with abnormal psychometric scores may be predisposed to developing IBS following an infectious gastroenteritis.)

Klein KB. Controlled treatment trials in the irritable bowel syndrome: A critique. Gastroenterology 1988;95:232–241. (A comprehensive critique of controlled treatment trials in IBS up to 1988. The author concludes that because of significant methodologic problems in all published trials, no pharmacological treatment has been shown to improve IBS symptoms.)

Manning AP, Thompson WD, Heaton KW. Towards positive diagnosis in the irritable bowel syndrome. BMJ 1978;2:653–654. (The first study to show symptoms to occur more commonly in

IBS patients than patients with other gastrointestinal diseases or normal subjects. These six symptoms have since become known as the Manning Criteria for IBS.)

Mertz H, Naliboff B, Munakata J, et al. Altered rectal perception is a biological marker of patients with the irritable bowel syndrome. Gastroenterology 1995;109:40–52. (Almost all patients with IBS in this study had some evidence for altered rectal perception in the form of lowered thresholds for discomfort, increased intensity of sensations, or altered viscerosomatic referral patterns. This study suggests that IBS patients have rectal "hypersensitivity," which may contribute to their symptoms.)

Munakata J, Naliboff B, Harraf F, et al. Repetitive sigmoid stimulation induces rectal hyperalgesia in patients with irritable syndrome. Gastroenterology 1997;112:55–63. (Splanchnic afferents stimulation by repetitive balloon distention in the sigmoid colon in patients with IBS caused a lowering of thresholds and altered abdominal referral patterns during rectal balloon distention. This study suggests that IBS patients may be more susceptible to central sensitization than normal subjects.)

Silverman DH, Munakata JA, Ennes H, et al. Regional cerebral activity in normal and pathological perception of visceral pain. Gastroenterology 1997;112:64–72. (Patients with IBS showed a lack of anterior cingulate cortex activation and significant increase in activation of the left prefrontal cortex in response to painful rectal balloon distention or the anticipation of painful rectal balloon distention using Positron Emission Tomography (PET). This study suggests that IBS patients have abnormal brain activation in response to visceral pain.)

Talley NJ, Owen BK, Boyce P, et al. Psychological treatments for irritable syndrome: a critique of controlled treatment trials. American Journal of Gastroenterology 1996;91:277–283. (A comprehensive critique of psychological treatment trials in patients with IBS. The authors conclude that the efficacy of psychological treatment in IBS has not been definitely established because of methodologic inadequacies of studies performed to date.)

Talley NJ, Zinsmeister AR, Melton III LJ. Irritable bowel syndrome in a community: symptom subgroups, risk factors, and health care utilization. Am J Epidemiol 1995;142:76–83. (Approximately 23% of respondents to a questionnaire survey over the age of 60 reported the initial onset of IBS symptoms during the previous year compared with 10% of young respondents. This suggests that elderly people develop IBS symptoms more commonly than previously thought.)

Chapter 4

EMERGING THERAPIES FOR HEPATITIS C

Geetanjali A. Akerkar, MD, and Teresa L. Wright, MD

BACKGROUND

Approximately 1.8% of the population are hepatitis C positive, which is a total of 3.9 million cases of hepatitis C in the United States. The prevalence rate rises dramatically from children to young adults, and most patients who have hepatitis C are between 30 and 39 years of age. Intravenous drug use is the greatest risk factor associated with acute hepatitis C infection and accounts for 53% of all new cases. Other high-risk behaviors account for 25% of cases; these include needle-stick transmission (5%), multiple sex partners (5%), household contacts (5%), and blood transfusions (3%). Infection with the hepatitis C virus falls slightly below alcoholism as a cause of cirrhosis, end-stage liver disease, and hepatocellular carcinoma, all of which result in more than 8000 deaths annually.

Chronic hepatitis C infection is often silent and discovered only by routine biochemical testing. Symptoms are typically absent, and only 25% of patients with post-transfusion hepatitis develop jaundice. Fulminant or subacute liver failure with the hepatitis C virus is rare. Approximately 33% of patients with chronic infection have normal or minimally elevated transaminase levels. However, some patients may have significant histologic changes despite normal aminotransferase concentration, and some present with advanced liver disease complicated by variceal bleeding, ascites, coagulopathy, or encephalopathy. The mean interval between exposure to the virus and development of chronic hepatitis, cirrhosis, and hepatocellular carcinoma is estimated to be 15 years, 20 years, and 30 years, respectively. Discussion of the natural history of infection is summarized in Figure 4.1. Hepatitis C has also been associated with several hepatic and extra-hepatic syndromes including porphyria cutanea tarda, Mooren's ulcers, type II cryoglobulinemia, and membranoproliferative glomerulonephritis.

Given the high morbidity and mortality rates associated with

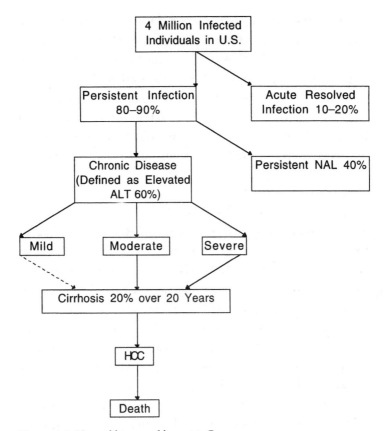

Figure 4.1. Natural history of hepatitis C

hepatitis C infection, the goal of treatment is to eradicate the hepatitis C virus early in the course of disease to prevent progression to end-stage liver disease. However, no drug has been effective in consistently eradicating hepatitis C infection in patients.

It is therefore important to determine which patients with hepatitis C should receive therapy and to identify those patients in whom response is so low that a therapeutic trial should not be given. Guidelines need to be established for discontinuation of initial therapy in patients who are unlikely to benefit. Retreatment of patients who do not respond to therapy and treatment regimens in patients in whom therapy is slowly becoming effective need to be assessed. Also, the optimal duration of treatment in patients who respond initially needs further clarification. Finally, we need to consider the role of combination therapy and whether it should be initiated early in the treatment regimen or be reserved for refractory cases. This chapter reviews treatment trials and strategies aimed at improving response rates in patients.

VIROLOGY

The hepatitis C virus is a positive-strand RNA virus related to the Flaviviridae family. The hepatitis C genome, which is 9400 nucleotides in length, encodes a polypeptide consisting of structural and nonstructural domains. Like many RNA viruses, hepatitis C virus has an inherently high mutation rate that results in considerable heterogeneity throughout the genome. There are nine major types of hepatitis C virus with sequence homology varying from 66 to 69% between genotypes and 40 different subtypes with 77 to 79% homology between subtypes. The 5'-untranslated region contains a highly conserved region that has a 92% homology among different hepatitis C genotypes. Quasi species are closely related, yet heterogeneous sequences of hepatitis C virus, which result from mutations occurring during viral replication, have been found in infected patients. Type 1 hepatitis C virus is the most prevalent genotype in the United States and is present in approximately 65% of infected patients.

The mechanism of persistence and cellular injury by hepatitis C virus is not well characterized. Persistence appears to result from the ability of the virus to replicate with a high rate of mutation, which leads to a series of quasi species that allow the virus to escape immunologic surveillance. The severity of disease in patients results from an interplay of many variables including viral load, genotype, host immune response to infection, and environmental factors such as alcohol.

INTERFERON TREATMENT

Interferon (IFN) has been studied in the treatment of patients with non-A, non-B hepatitis and, more recently, hepatitis C. Two recombinant α IFNs, IFN-α-2b and -2a, are FDA-approved as initial therapy in patients with chronic hepatitis C infection. Three million units (MU) of IFN-α-2b administered subcutaneously three times a week for 6 months was approved in 1991, and 3 MU of IFN-α-2a administered subcutaneously three times a week for 12 months was approved in 1996. IFNs are a family of intracellular proteins that have established antiviral and immunomodulatory properties. They bind to specific cell surface receptors, activating various enzymes and genes that affect viral replication, uncoating, assembly, and cell entry. IFNs also increase natural killer cell activity, enhance maturation of cytotoxic T cells, and increase cell surface expression of class I histocompatibility leukocyte antigens (HLAs), thereby promoting immune clearance of infected hepatocytes. Other IFNs studied in the treatment of patients with hepatitis C include consensus IFN (CIFN), leukocyte-derived IFN, and several IFN-β products.

Initial randomized controlled trials on IFN performed in the United States and Europe evaluated the safety profiles and efficacy rates of 3 MU of subcutaneous therapy three times a week for 6 months. Response, which was defined as normalization of serum alanine aminotransferase (ALT) levels at the end of treatment, approached 50%. However, relapse rates were high (70% after an initial course of therapy) with long-term sustained response (defined as normal ALT levels and absent hepatitis C RNA for at least 6 months of therapy) achievable in approximately 15% of patients.

IFN-α is associated with several side effects including flu-like symptoms, which occur within 6 to 8 hours of initiation of treatment, and are experienced in the majority of patients. Other side effects include nausea, headache, fever, myalgia, and arthralgia. However, side effects are usually tolerable at doses of 3 to 6 MU of IFN-α, and tachyphylaxis generally develops quickly. Other side effects develop after several days and include fatigue, leukopenia, thrombocytopenia, alopecia, irritability, and depression. Thyroid abnormalities have also been noted. A temporary decrease in dosage is required in some patients usually because of transient leukopenia and thrombocytopenia. IFN-α has also been reported to aggravate liver disease in patients with autoimmune hepatitis who are erroneously diagnosed with chronic hepatitis C. Therefore, the diagnosis of hepatitis C must be confirmed with a recombinant immunoblot assay in patients without an identified risk factor for hepatitis C infection.

A number of investigators have sought to identify factors associated with response and explore different dosages and duration of treatment because of the low sustained virologic and biochemical response rates in patients treated with 3 MU IFN-α-2b three times a week for 6 months.

PREDICTORS OF RESPONSE

Favorable clinical predictors of response include mild to moderate liver inflammation, absence of cirrhosis, short disease duration, low body weight, and decreased hepatic iron content. Viral specific factors associated with an improved response rate include a genotype other than type 1, low serum and hepatic hepatitis C RNA levels, minimal genetic diversity of hepatitis C, and lack of anti-hepatitis C immunoglobin M (IgM) core antibodies. Multivariate analyses have provided estimates of which features are independent predictors for a long-term response to therapy in patients. In large trials, the two most important independent predictors have been hepatitis C RNA levels and viral genotype. However, the genotype rather than viral load has been more strongly associated with response in several large studies. The endpoints of these trials are not consistent. Biochemical and histologic response can be achieved and occasionally sustained after therapy despite the low-level persistence of hepatitis C RNA and, conversely, relapse may occur occasionally despite a transiently negative result on polymerase chain reaction (PCR) after treatment. Although numerous pretreatment characteristics are hypothesized to be independently associated with response to IFN treatment, these factors have not been validated in a prospective study. The accuracy of these predictive factors in correctly identifying response or nonresponse during treatment is only 57%, 58%, and 61% for hepatitis C RNA levels, viral genotype, and cirrhosis, respectively. Physicians should not risk excluding patients because of strict pretreatment criteria; the positive predictive value of these pretreatment criteria remains questionable.

MEASUREMENT OF RESPONSE

Response to treatment is measured at the end of treatment and during the follow-up period. Sustained response is defined as an end-treatment biochemical and virologic response followed by normal ALT levels and indistinguishable hepatitis C RNA levels during follow-up. During therapy, the ALT values follow one of four general patterns: ALT levels normalize and remain normal throughout the follow-up period (sustained response), ALT levels normalize during therapy but then become abnormal after termination of therapy (relapse), ALT levels become temporarily normal and then abnormal again during treatment (breakthrough), and the ALT levels remain abnormal throughout the course of therapy (nonresponder) (Fig 4.2).

A. Sustained Response to Therapy

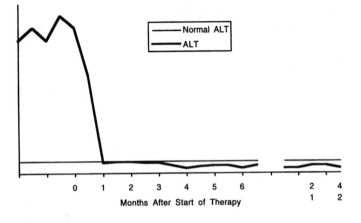

B. Relapse After Discontinuation of Therapy

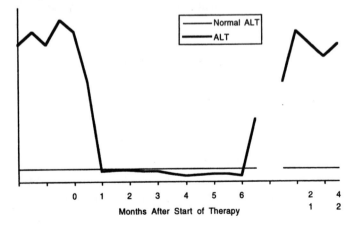

Figure 4.2. A. Chronic hepatitis C—sustained response to therapy
B. Chronic hepatitis C—relapse after discontinuation of therapy

C. Transient Partial Response to Therapy

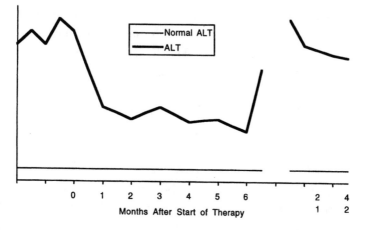

D No Response to Therapy

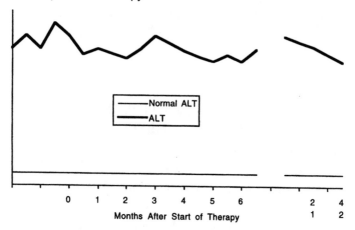

Figure 4.2. —*continued*
C. Chronic hepatitis C—transient partial response to therapy
D. Chronic hepatitis C—no response to therapy (Reprinted with
permission from Hoofnagle J, Di Bisceglie A. The treatment of Chronic
Viral Hepatitis. N Engl J Med 1997;336:347–356.)

The endpoints of successful therapy are in constant evolution. Patients with normal aminotransferase concentrations have significant histologic findings. Conversely, several studies have noted an improvement in hepatic histology in patients who did not normalize aminotransferases on therapy. The significance of this finding remains unclear. The discrepancy between biochemical and histologic responses to therapy has resulted in the measurement of hepatitis C RNA levels because a decrease in a hepatitis C RNA level may correlate with improved liver histology.

At this time, the optimal goal of therapy is the achievement of sustained normalization of ALT levels, clearance of hepatitis C RNA, and improvement in liver histology. Long-term follow-up of patients who experienced a sustained response to IFN therapy indicates that more than 90% of patients will maintain normal ALT levels and nondeductibility of hepatitis C RNA over 1 to 6 years of follow-up. Histologic activity markedly improves in such patients. Whether this represents effective treatment is uncertain. However, it is believed that histologic improvement will lead to improved survival rates, although this assumption has not been supported by data.

RECENT STRATEGIES TO IMPROVE RESPONSE

Investigators have sought to improve sustained biochemical and virologic response rates by increasing the dose and duration of IFN therapy. Researchers have found that a high initial dose of 6 MU with tapering on the basis of biochemical response compared with a dose of 3 MU for 12 months resulted in a higher sustained response rate even in patients with genotype 1B. Other researchers have noted that increasing the dose to 3 MU at week 12 in patients who do not respond to treatment results in response in a small percentage of patients. These findings are not universal. Some researchers have been unable to demonstrate an effect of increasing the dose on overall rate of response.

A recent meta-analysis of 33 trials comparing patients who were administered 3 MU to 6 MU of IFN found higher doses improved sustained biochemical response by a mean of 17% (p<.001). However, a significant increase in side effects was also noted in patients who were administered the higher dose, and these side effects forced researchers to decrease the dose in many patients. In addition, a significant duration effect was noted. Three MU for 12 months versus 6 months improved biochemical response rates associated with a higher sustained response rate of a mean increase of 16% (p<.001). A mean increase in response rate of 20% (p =.003) was noted in patients who were administered 6 MU of IFN. Researchers decided the best efficacy and risk ratio was treatment of 3 MU of IFN three times a week for at least 12 months. Similarly, other investigators have found that treatment for 18 months at a dose of 3 MU produced improved histological and biochemical response rates in patients when compared with shorter regimens.

DIFFERENT TYPES OF INTERFERON

IFNs are a family of naturally occurring small proteins that are produced and secreted by cells in response to viral infections. IFN-α and -β are classified as type 1 IFNs, which include more than 25 different molecules. Consensus IFN is a new recombinant type 1 IFN containing 166 amino acids. CIFN was derived by scanning the sequences of several natural α IFNs and assigning the most frequently observed amino acid in each corresponding position. In vitro, CIFN displays five to ten times higher biological activity than naturally occurring type 1 IFNs. A recent large randomized, double-blind, controlled study of 704 IFN-naive patients found comparable initial and sustained response between the two groups but found that patients treated with 9 ug of CIFN had a significantly greater mean decrease in hepatitis C RNA levels at the end of treatment compared to patients treated with 3 MU of IFN-α-2b for a 24-week period. ($P = .037$) In a subgroup analysis, hepatitis C RNA response at the end of treatment in patients with genotype 1 was better after CIFN treatment when compared with those patients who had received IFN-α-2b treatment. Patients who did not respond or relapsed after treatment with either IFN-α 2b or CIFN were treated with a higher dose of CIFN, which was 15 ug for a 24-week period. Sustained virologic response was found in 32% of patients who relapse compared with 8% of patients who do not respond to treatment. In summary, studies of CIFN show comparable initial and sustained responses to other IFNα treatment, and CIFN may have an advantage over other IFNs in the treatment of genotype 1 infection in patients.

IFN-α n1 is produced from a human lymphoid cell line and consists of multiple IFN-α subtypes of which at least two are glycosylated. This differs from the recombinant IFNs, which are unglycosylated proteins. Comparison of IFN-α-n1 treatment with IFN-α-2a and -2b treatment has found that it is just as efficacious as the recombinant products and may offer lower rates of post-treatment relapse. In addition, in a large multicenter trial, prolongation of therapy to 12 months was superior to 6 months of therapy in achieving biochemical and virologic response; however, this observation will need further study.

TREATMENT WITH RIBAVIRIN

New drugs are being investigated to improve response rates because only approximately 20% of patients treated with IFN achieve sustained response. Ribavirin is a guanosine analogue with broad spectrum activity against several RNA and DNA viruses including the flavivirus family. Ribavirin can be administered orally and is usually well-tolerated by patients. The exact mechanism of action is unknown, but it is speculated that ribavirin may inhibit viral dependent RNA polymerases and may also serve as an inhibitor of macrophage pro-inflammatory cytokines. Monotherapy with ribavirin is not an effective antiviral treatment against hepatitis C. Ribavirin treatment at a dose of 600 mg two times a day for 12 months resulted in a biochemical and histologic response without an associated decrease in hepatitis C RNA levels in small placebo-controlled trials. These effects were also not sustained when ribavirin therapy was discontinued. Hemolysis necessitating a dose decrease has been seen in 13% of patients. Other side effects include fatigue, depression, insomnia, anorexia, nausea, and rash.

Combination therapy can be effective in improving response rates and minimizing drug resistance in patients. Initial pilot studies reported sustained normalization of aminotransferase levels associated with a decrease in hepatitis C RNA levels in 40% of patients in the combination therapy group compared with none in the IFN group (p<.05). Up to 80% of patients who relapsed and 10 to 25% of patients who did not respond to previous IFN therapy had a sustained biochemical and virologic response, although the number of patients studied in these groups is small. In patients who are IFN-naive, sustained virologic response occurred in 45% of patients in the combination group versus 23% in the IFN group (p<.05). In a long-term follow-up study, nearly 50% of patients treated with ribavirin and IFN-α-2a for a 24-week period achieved biochemical and virologic response for at least 2 years after termination of therapy. Many questions however are still unanswered. Should combination therapy be used in IFN-naive patients or be reserved for patients who do not respond to treatment or patients who relapse? What is the optimal dose and duration of combination therapy? There are ongoing multi-center trials that will answer some of these questions in the upcoming years.

NEW THERAPIES

There have been reports of several promising agents for the treatment of patients with hepatitis C. Studies to date have been small. Pentoxifylline in addition to IFN-α-2b improved initial biochemical response rates to therapy. However, no sustained benefit was noted. In patients who showed either no response to IFN or only partial response, ursodeoxycholic acid in addition to IFN significantly improved the biochemical response rates compared with IFN alone, but no parallel improvement in hepatitis C RNA levels were noted. Similarly, granulocyte-macrophage colony-stimulation factor (GM-CSF) administered in combination with IFN in IFN-resistant patients resulted in an improved biochemical response but had no effect on viral load. Finally phlebotomy followed by IFN retreatment in patients who did not respond to previous IFN therapy resulted in a decrease in serum ALT and hepatitis C RNA levels and no improvement in liver histology. Low hepatic iron content has been associated with an improved sustained response rate. The long-term benefit of all of these treatments remains to be seen, and these therapeutic approaches should be reserved for controlled clinical trials.

RETREATMENT IN PATIENTS WHO RELAPSE AND PATIENTS WHO DO NOT RESPOND TO TREATMENT

A review of the data on 11 reports of approximately 500 patients who did not respond to treatment found no significant differences in obtaining an initial response or a sustained response with retreatment with standard therapy of 3 MU of IFN for 6 months compared with higher doses or longer duration. Also, no difference was recorded comparing different types of IFN.

However, results of retreatment in patients who responded but relapsed are quite different. A total of 527 patients were reviewed in 10 publications. Patients were initially treated with 3 MU of IFN for 6 months. Comparison of retreatment rates for 6 months versus 12 months showed a sustained response rate of 16.9% compared with 51%, respectively. No differences in response rates were noted using different types or doses of IFN. Some investigators have found that long-term maintenance therapy at a dose of 1 MU of IFN three times a week resulted in prolonged normal liver test results in patients who had previously relapsed. However, viremia resurfaced in some patients. Maintenance therapy is an attractive option, but it is still unclear whether maintenance therapy will provide long-term benefit in improving the natural history of hepatitis C and reducing mortality in patients.

In summary, retreatment with IFN should be reserved for patients who show complete biochemical and virologic response but relapse after termination of therapy. These should be retreated for 12 months with hopes of achieving a sustained response rate in 40 to 60% of patients. Promising results with CIFN and ribavirin in patients who did not respond to treatment and particularly in patients who relapsed suggest that these drugs may play a future role in the treatment of this group of patients. Patient groups who may benefit from treatment are summarized in Table 4.1.

Table 4.1

INDICATIONS FOR RETREATMENT WITH INTERFERON THERAPY[a]

Treatment Indicated	Treatment is Controversial or Experimental	Treatment Contraindicated
Previously untreated patients with abnormal ALT levels	Patients with persistently normal ALT levels	Patients with active substance abuse
Patients who relapsed	Liver transplant recipients	Patients with major depressive illness
Patients with acute infection	Patients with compensated cirrhosis	Patients with decompensated liver disease
Patients at high risk of cirrhosis	Patients age < 18 years	Renal transplant recipients
Patients with extra-hepatic manifestations such as cryoglobunemia	Patients with membranoproliferative glomerulonephritis	Patients with autoimmune liver disease
		Pregnant patients
		Patients with lymphopenia or thrombocytopenia
		Patients with untreated thyroid disease
		Patients who previously did not respond to interferon therapy

[a]*Therapy should not be limited by patient mode of infection with hepatitis C, HIV status, hepatitis C RNA levels, or genotype.*
ALT = *alanine aminotransferase.*

THERAPY FOR ATYPICAL FORMS OF CHRONIC HEPATITIS C

ACUTE HEPATITIS C INFECTION

Patients with acute hepatitis C infection have been treated with IFN-α in an attempt to lower the rate of persistent infection, which can be as high as 85%. Small randomized controlled trials found that therapy with IFN-α was effective treatment of hepatitis C RNA and decreased ALT levels in 39 to 90% of patients. In the same recent meta-analysis described above that compared eight trials, the sustained ALT response rate at 12 months was 53% in the treated group versus 32% in the control group ($P = .02$). The hepatitis C virus clearance rate at the end of treatment was 41% versus 4% in the control group ($P < .001$). These findings suggest that therapy during acute infection is effective and should be initiated.

TREATMENT OF PATIENTS WITH NORMAL ALT LEVELS

A large percentage of patients with chronic hepatitis C infection have normal ALT levels and no symptoms of chronic liver disease. Pilot studies in these patients have found that few have long-term responses to treatment. Surprisingly, investigators have found that the mean level of hepatitis C RNA was not different between subjects with normal ALT levels and those with increased ALT levels. In addition, studies of hepatitis C genotypes have shown no difference in the distribution of different genotypes between the two groups. These findings are, however, controversial because some investigators report an increased proportion of genotype 2 in patients with normal ALT levels. Only 27% of patients were found to have normal liver histology in a recent review of liver histology in patients with normal ALT levels. In addition, 19% of patients were found to have chronic hepatitis with moderate activity. Fibrosis is usually absent, but cirrhosis has been observed. The poor response rate in treatment of patients with IFN may be the result of viral diversity with an increase in the number of quasi species. The long-term outcome of patients with normal ALT levels is unknown and needs to be studied further.

TREATMENT OF PATIENTS WITH CIRRHOSIS

The 5-year survival rate of patients with Child's C cirrhosis is estimated to be 91%. Hepatic decompensation occurs in 18% of patients with Child's C cirrhosis and the development of hepatocellular carcinoma occurs in 7% of patients at 5 years. Sustained response rates in patients with cirrhosis are 9 to 16%, and these rates are considerably lower compared with rates in noncirrhotic individuals. As mentioned earlier, cirrhosis in patients is an independent predictor of poor response rates. However, in a large prospective trial of 90 patients with compensated cirrhosis, treatment with IFN-α (6 MU three times a week for 12 to 24 weeks) resulted in improved liver function and a reduced risk of hepatocellular carcinoma. The benefit was most marked in the patients in whom a sustained remission is induced (two patients in the treated group compared with 17 patients in the control group, $P = .002$). In contrast, a large European trial failed to show the same benefit when adjusted for the fact the patients in the control group were significantly older and had more severe liver disease than those in the treated group. In a more recent trial, the sustained response rate was 21% with combination therapy with ribavirin and IFN, which is significantly higher than rates in patients treated with IFN alone. Information on IFN treatment in patients with decompensated cirrhosis is limited since these patients are typically excluded from randomized trials.

Further investigation is warranted given the significant benefit in reducing the risk of HCC in patients with compensated cirrhosis, which is seen in at least one prospective trial of IFN. Mortality from disease is an easily measured endpoint in this patient population. This contrasts to patients with minimal disease in whom progression to death takes many decades.

HUMAN IMMUNODEFICIENCY VIRUS AND HEPATITIS C VIRUS

The prevalence of coinfection with HIV and hepatitis C virus is high in hemophiliacs and other patients who acquire their infection from blood contact. In patients with intact immunity systems, chronic viral hepatitis is typically a disease that progresses slowly over several decades although some patients have rapid progression to end-stage liver disease. Several studies have evaluated the natural history of hepatitis C in patients with HIV infection and found that HIV coinfection accelerates the course of liver disease. Liver failure was significantly higher in the coinfected population. Two small studies have shown that treatment with IFN in patients with HIV and hepatitis C coinfection results in decreased hepatitis C RNA rates and improvement in histology. Historically, aggressive treatment of hepatitis C in patients who were HIV-positive was not recommended since HIV, not hepatitis C, was believed to determine life expectancy. Availability of effective HIV anti-retrovirals is changing the natural history of HIV infection, such that aggressive treatment of hepatitis C infection may be warranted in the future.

HEPATITIS C INFECTION IN THE TRANSPLANT SETTING

The mean prevalence of hepatitis C RNA by PCR was 2.4% in a national study of 3078 cadaver organ donors. Approximately 48% of organ recipients from anti-hepatitis C positive donors develop post-transplantation liver disease. In addition, hepatitis C cirrhosis is one of the leading indications for orthotropic liver transplantation in the United States.

Recurrent infection is almost universal, and more than 95% of patients with pretransplantation infection have post-transplantation persistent viremia. Recurrent infection is defined as abnormal serum aminotransferase levels and, more importantly, abnormal liver histology. Despite the high recurrence rate, the reported 5-year survival rate is approximately 75%. Recurrent infection is required to initiate therapy in most series. Small studies have found 12 to 28% of liver transplant recipients treated with IFN for 6 months have a biochemical response that is defined as normalization of aminotransferase. However, there is a small risk of rejection induced by IFN treatment. Longer duration of therapy improved sustained response rates in immunocompetent individuals. Two pilot studies have shown that treatment with 800 to 1200 mg daily of ribavirin for 3 months resulted in normalization of ALT levels, but relapse was common. Hepatitis C RNA levels decreased, but the virus remained detectable and liver histology did not improve. Combination therapy with IFN and ribavirin for 6 months has showed biochemical and histologic response. These studies are small and need to be confirmed in larger trials. Although treatment results in biochemical and virologic response, treatment has not been shown to improve graft and patient survival. There have been reports of early graft loss in renal transplant patients undergoing IFN treatment. Treatment should be considered only in patients with viremia and liver injury documented by histology. Ribavirin has been used to treat four patients receiving bone marrow transplantation during and after transplantation. Two of these patients became hepatitis C negative at 12 month follow-up. These results are preliminary and warrant further investigation.

TREATMENT OF PATIENTS WITH GLOMERULONEPHRITIS

Hepatitis C virus is associated with several extra-hepatic syndromes including cryoglobulinemia as mentioned previously. Renal disease, namely membranoproliferative glomerulonephritis, develops in approximately 50% of patients. Small case studies have found that treatment with IFN-α for 6 to 12 months results in a significant decrease in proteinuria but no improvement in renal function. However, relapse of viremia and renal disease was common after completion of therapy. In contrast, 53 patients with type II cryoglobulinemia were treated with 1.5 MU of IFN-α-2a for 1 week followed by 3 MU for 23 weeks in a large prospective study, and patients treated with IFN had a significant decrease in creatinine ($P = .006$) compared with controls. However, relapse was common. It remains to be seen whether treatment with IFN will have any long-term effect on renal function.

SUMMARY

We have reviewed treatment trials and strategies aimed at improving primary and sustained response rates in patients with chronic hepatitis C infection. It is important to note that all studies report short-term benefit measured by either biochemical, virologic, or histologic parameters. There has been no study to date showing the beneficial effect of any drug on endpoints such as mortality. It is unclear whether treatment affects morbidity rates of chronic disease because of the numerous side effects associated with therapy. Large prospective long-term studies are needed to evaluate the benefit of therapy on morbidity and mortality rates in patients with chronic hepatitis C infection before a standard treatment modality is established.

SUGGESTED READINGS

Dove L, Wright T. Hepatitis/HIV coinfection-infection with hepatitis viruses in patients with human immunodeficiency virus: medical dilemma or inconsequential coincidence? Advances in Gastroenterology, Hepatology and Clinical Nutrition 1996;1:231–239. (This article offers a comprehensive review of the natural history and therapeutic options for patients coinfected with HIV and hepatitis C.)

Hoofnagle J, Di Bisceglie A. The treatment of Chronic Viral Hepatitis. N Engl J Med 1997;336: 347–356. (This reference offer an excellent overview of treatment strategies for patients with hepatitis C infection.)

Johnson R, Gretch D, Couser W, et al. Hepatitis C virus-associated glomerulonephritis. Kidney Int 1994;46:1700–1704. (This article provides a good overview of the benefits and limitations of treatment of patients with renal disease and Hepatitis C.)

NIH Consensus Development Conference on Management of Hepatitis C. Hepatology 1997;26(Suppl):2s–10s. (This reference offers an excellent overview of treatment strategies for patients with hepatitis C infection.)

Pessoa M, Wright T. Hepatitis C infection in Transplantation. Clinics in Liver Disease 1997;1:663–690. (This reference outlines key points regarding the transmission of chronic hepatitis C infection, treatment of patients with chronic hepatitis C infection, and role of transplantation in patients with chronic hepatitis C infection.)

Poynard T, Leroy V, CoHard M, et al. Meta-analysis of interferon randomized trial in the treatment of hepatitis C. Hepatology 1996:778–789. (This meta-analysis offers an excellent summary of the trials on IFN therapy to date.)

Chapter 5

COLORECTAL CANCER AND POLYP SURVEILLANCE

John H. Bond, MD

DEFINITION: SCREENING
VERSUS SURVEILLANCE

Screening for colorectal cancer usually involves simple, inexpensive, often indirect tests designed to identify asymptomatic, average-risk individuals who have an increased likelihood of early colorectal cancer or a clinically significant adenomatous polyp (adenoma). Current evidence-based practice guidelines recommend annual fecal occult blood testing (FOBT) plus flexible sigmoidoscopy approximately every 5 years for asymptomatic patients older than 50 years of age who do not have additional risk factors for the disease. It increasingly has been recognized, however, that some patients are at higher risk for developing colorectal neoplasia and may benefit from periodic complete structural examination of the large bowel rather than just undergoing screening tests. This approach to above average-risk patients is usually referred to as surveillance, not screening. This chapter discusses several special risk factors that help identify patients likely to benefit from surveillance and reviews the surveillance recommendations contained in recently developed or revised guidelines.

RISK FACTORS FOR COLORECTAL CANCER

Most people—approximately 70 million in the United States—are at average risk for colorectal cancer because they are more than 50 years of age, which is the time in life when the incidence of the disease begins to increase appreciably. Several above average or high-risk groups have been identified and include the following: patients with a family history of colorectal cancer or adenomatous polyps, patients with a personal history of successful resection of colorectal cancer or adenomatous polyps, and patients with long-standing chronic ulcerative colitis or Crohn's colitis. Depending on several clinical variables, the risk of developing colorectal cancer in many patients in these high-risk groups is sufficient to justify periodic definitive surveillance examination of the entire large bowel rather than routine screening.

SURVEILLANCE METHODS

Colonoscopy is the procedure of choice for surveillance of patients with colorectal neoplasia. Colonoscopy is more accurate than air-contrast barium enema for the detection of small polypoid lesions. The entire large bowel can be thoroughly examined with a single examination by experienced endoscopists with minimal risk and discomfort in more than 95% of patients. Most importantly, colonoscopy allows the immediate biopsy of suspicious lesions and resection of most detected polyps in a single sitting with a single bowel preparation.

Although the alternative surveillance strategy of performing barium enema plus flexible sigmoidoscopy may be initially less expensive than performing primary colonoscopy, the need to perform subsequent colonoscopy anyway for all patients found to have an abnormality makes this approach, on average, almost equal in cost. The complication rate for colonoscopy, although higher than that of barium enema, is currently very low. Major complications of perforation or bleeding occur in approximately 0.1% of cases performed by experienced physicians. Most of these major complications result from polypectomy rather than from purely diagnostic examinations, so they perhaps are more justified on a risk/benefit basis.

FAMILY HISTORY OF
COLORECTAL NEOPLASIA

A family history of colorectal cancer or adenomas identifies patients who are at higher risk for colorectal cancer and may require monitoring (Table 5.1). Three patterns of inherited

Table 5.1

ENDOSCOPIC SURVIELLANCE FOR PATIENTS WITH
FAMILIAL RISK FOR COLORECTAL CANCER

Risk	Test	Interval	Age To Begin
FAP [a]	Sigmoidoscopy	6 to 12 month	10 to 12 years
HPNCC [b]	Colonoscopy	2 year	25 years
Low familial risk for sporadic cancer	FOBT Sigmoidoscopy	Annual 5 year	40 years
High familial risk for sporadic cancer	Colonoscopy	5 year	40 years

[a] *Identified by family history and genetic testing*
[b] *Identified by family history ("Amsterdam criteria") and genetic testing*
FAP = familial adenomatous polyposts; FOBT = fecal occult blood test; HPNCC = hereditary nonpolyposis colorectal cancer.

risk have been defined. The familial adenomatous polyposis (FAP) syndromes make up less than 1% of all colorectal cancers, and hereditary nonpolyposis colorectal cancer
(HNPCC) syndromes account for approximately 6%. Recent
studies also indicate that a sizable percentage (50% or more)
of "sporadic" cancers may also have an underlying inherited
genetic cause.

FAP results from the autosomal dominant inheritance of a
mutated adenomatous polyposis coli (APC) gene on chromosome 5. Affected patients develop hundreds to thousands of
colorectal adenomas. The average patient age of adenoma detection is 16 years, and virtually all affected patients develop
colorectal carcinoma by 45 years of age. Although cancer risk
correlates with polyp count and age, approximately 7% of
patients develop cancer by 21 years of age. Extracolonic adenomas are also common, especially in the periampullary area of
the duodenum, and may undergo malignant transformation later
in life. Patients with a family history of FAP should be offered
genetic testing and counseling at 10 to 12 years of age. Annual
or biannual flexible sigmoidoscopy is recommended for patients
who test positive, and prophylactic colectomy is indicated when
adenomas begin to appear. Periodic upper endoscopy surveil-

lance every 1 to 3 years, depending on findings, helps protect patients against duodenal carcinomas.

HNPCC syndromes (Lynch syndromes I and II) results from autosomal dominantly inherited mutations of one of four DNA mismatch repair genes on chromosomes 2, 3, or 7. Products of these genes normally help repair spontaneously occurring errors in DNA nucleotide replication. Loss of this function leads to genomic instability, which makes the epithelial cells more prone to other acquired genetic changes that promote rapid neoplasia development. Colorectal cancers occur at an earlier age, are preceded by the development of several polyps, and are more often located in the right colon. Multiple synchronous and metachronous cancers are common. Although these cancers often have unfavorable histologic features, stage-specific survival in patients is actually better than that of patients with sporadic cancers. Endometrial and other extraintestinal cancers are common in some families (Lynch Syndrome II). Affected families are identified by pedigree analysis. According to the Amsterdam Criteria for identifying families with HNPCC, the syndrome is likely present if three first-degree relatives have colorectal cancer for at least two generations and one relative was diagnosed before 50 years of age. Genetic tests to identify affected members within a family are emerging. Colonoscopy every 1 to 2 years beginning at 20 to 25 years of age and pelvic surveillance of women in selected kindreds are recommended for family members who have likely inherited the genetic abnormality.

Familial clustering of sporadic colorectal cancers and adenomas is common even when the hereditary syndromes of FAP and HNPCC are ruled out. The relative risk of colorectal cancer in first-degree relatives (i.e, siblings, parents, and children) of patients with this cancer is two- to fourfold. Pedigree and endoscopic studies implicate a partially penetrant, autosomally dominant genetic predisposition to colorectal cancer. Risk is related to the number of family members with colorectal cancer, younger age at diagnosis, and perhaps to the occurrence of right-sided cancers. Screening and surveillance are stratified according to assessed risk. Patients with high familial risk (i.e., a first-degree relative diagnosed with colorectal cancer at a young age or two or more affected relatives) should undergo colonoscopy every 5 years beginning at 40 years of age. Patients with lower risk (i.e., one first-degree relative with colorectal cancer diagnosed at an advanced age) should undergo standard screening with FOBT and flexible sigmoidoscopy beginning at 40 years of age.

A recent analysis of data collected by the National Polyp Study, which was a multicenter trial of postpolypectomy surveillance, indicates that relatives of patients who have undergone colonoscopic resection of adenomatous polyps may also have a risk of subsequent colorectal cancer that is sufficient to justify surveillance. Two clinical situations identify individuals who have substantial risk: (1) siblings of patients with adenomas that are detected before 60 years of age and (2) siblings of patients with adenomas detected at any age if a parent also had a history of colorectal cancer. The high-risk relatives of patients with adenomas should also be offered surveillance colonoscopy every 5 years beginning at 40 years of age.

POSTPOLYPECTOMY SURVEILLANCE

Some patients who had successful colonoscopic resection of one or more adenomatous polyps have an increased risk for recurrent adenomas and subsequent cancer and may benefit from long-term follow-up surveillance. Studies from St. Mark's Hospital in London and the Mayo Clinic show that patients with one small tubular adenoma found on proctosigmoidoscopy have no measurable increased subsequent risk of colorectal cancer. However, patients with large (more than 1 cm) or multiple adenomas or adenomas that contain villous tissue or high-grade dysplasia have a more than average likelihood of developing subsequent cancer unless careful follow-up colonoscopic surveillance is performed. Recent data from the National Polyp Study also indicate that a family history of colorectal cancer or adenoma increases the risk of subsequent cancer in patients who have been treated for polyps.

Pathologic studies and data from the National Polyp Study suggest that it takes, on the average, several years for a large adenoma to develop and grow and 8 to 12 years for a gross colorectal cancer to develop. Therefore, follow-up surveillance does not need to be performed frequently when accurate methods such as colonoscopy are employed. The purpose of surveillance is not just to find and resect small benign polyps; rather, it is to find and resect metachronous polyps before they grow to a clinically significant size at which they are more likely to undergo malignant degeneration.

The National Polyp Study determined colonoscopy performed 3 years after initial colonoscopic polypectomy detected clinically significant metachronous polyps as effectively as 1- and 3-year follow-up examinations. If no polyp was found on the first 3-year follow-up examination, little significant pathology was discovered on a second 3-year follow-up. Therefore, less frequent subsequent follow-up examinations are recommended for most patients. Widespread adoption of current follow-up surveillance guidelines will adequately protect this high-risk group while simultaneously appreciably decreasing the cost of surveillance programs.

The first surveillance colonoscopy should usually be performed 3 years after colonoscopic resection of large (more than 1 cm), multiple, or villous-containing adenomas (Table 5.2).

Table 5.2

ENDOSCOPIC SURVEILLANCE OF PATIENTS AFTER CURATIVE
RESECTION OF COLORECTAL CANCER OR ADVANCED POLYP

1. Administer initial colonoscopy to clear colon of synchronous neoplasia.
2. Perform surveillance colonoscopy in 3-year follow-up examination.
3. Increase patient follow-up intervals to every 5 years after a negative follow-up surveillance colonoscopy.
4. Perform flexible sigmoidoscopy every 3 to 6 months for 2 years after low anterior surgical resection of a Stage B or C rectosigmoid cancer.
5. Individualize patient follow-up schedule for age and comorbidity.

Because patients who have a single small tubular adenoma do not have an increased risk of cancer, follow-up surveillance may not be needed if the patients also do not have other risk factors such as a strong family history of large bowel neoplasia. Subsequent surveillance intervals can be safely increased to every 5 years after one negative 3-year follow-up colonoscopy. Surveillance should always be individualized according to the age and comorbidity of each patient and should be discontinued when it no longer is likely to be of benefit.

PATIENT SURVEILLANCE AFTER RESECTION OF COLORECTAL CANCER

The objectives of surveillance after curative resection of colorectal cancer are to detect treatable recurrences, missed synchronous cancer or adenomas, and subsequent metachronous neoplasia. Unfortunately, except for a small percentage of cases, curative treatment of recurrent cancer in patients is rarely possible, and palliation of unresectable recurrent cancer is not very effective. Furthermore, there is little evidence that palliative therapy is more effective when applied early in treatment compared to when recurrence causes obvious symptoms. The main objective of follow-up surveillance in most patients is to detect curable synchronous and metachronous cancer and adenomas.

Traditional follow-up strategies after colorectal cancer

surgery, which are still practiced in many centers, often consisted of too many tests that are performed too frequently and often for poorly defined reasons. Several outcome studies assessing the value of such conventional surveillance programs have concluded that survival rates and the detection of treatable recurrences are not substantially increased by this expensive rigorous approach. They concluded that intensive follow-up is not justified for most patients as long as effective treatment for recurrent or unresectable disease is lacking.

The incidence of synchronous cancers and polyps in patients with known cancer is 2 to 7% and 25 to 45%, respectively. Metachronous cancers and adenomas are reported in 2 to 5% and 20 to 40%, respectively. Follow-up examinations to detect metachronous neoplasia do not need to be frequent if accurate surveillance methods are employed since it takes 8 to 10 years for a neoplastic polyp to develop in a normal-appearing colon, grow to a clinically significant size, and degenerate into a cancer.

Based on available data, the following is a rational follow-up plan for patients after potentially curative resection of colorectal cancer (see Table 5.2):

1. Colonoscopy should be performed during the perioperative period (preferably before surgery so cancers and large polyps may be included in the resection) to clear the colon of synchronous neoplasia. If not feasible preoperatively because of an obstructing left colonic cancer, clearing colonoscopy is performed 3 to 6 months postoperatively if no distant metastases are found during surgery.

2. Postoperative visits are scheduled as needed to educate the patient about symptoms of early recurrence, check for postsurgical complications, and provide medical and emotional support.

3. Repeat colonoscopy is performed in 3 years, and, depending on findings, every 3 to 5 years thereafter.

4. Serial rectosigmoid examinations with flexible sigmoidoscopy are reserved for selected patients undergoing sphincter-sparing low anterior resections of rectosigmoid cancers.

Anastomotic (suture-line) recurrences of abdominal colon cancers (above the rectosigmoid colon) are rare with modern surgical techniques. In one large series of 1315 patients with such cancers, 2.7% of patients developed a possible anastomotic recurrence and resection of these lesions resulted in no long-term survivors. Thus, nearly all recurrences of proximal colonic cancer occur outside the bowel and rarely will be detected by follow-up surveillance examinations of the colon.

Local recurrences in the area of the anastomosis often occur after anterior resection of Dukes' B or C rectosigmoid cancers. These patients should be followed more closely with flexible sigmoidoscopy every 3 to 6 months for a period of at least 2 years because these recurrences may be amenable to radiation therapy and sometimes second surgical resections.

Long-term survival has been reported in patients undergoing surgical resection of solitary hepatic and, less often, pulmonary metastases. The literature dealing with surveillance for such potentially treatable recurrences is difficult to interpret because no uniform staging system is used, there are no prospective controls, and different survival endpoints are employed by different centers. Some reports indicate that approximately 30% of patients undergoing curative resection of colorectal cancer will develop apparent isolated hepatic metastases; approximately 25% of these patients will have metastases that will be resectable and have a 5-year survival rate of approximately 25%. Thus, the total number of patients with a favorable outcome is small and does not justify routine intensive surveillance for all postsurgical patients. Rather, selected patients who may be offered special intensive surveillance should be healthy enough to tolerate hepatic or pulmonary resections and have colorectal cancers with a substantial likelihood of metastasizing (Dukes' B or C).

Special intensive surveillance should usually not be prolonged beyond the first 2 years following colonic resection because the majority of solitary metastases occur during that time interval. Surveillance for this select group, which comprises 15 to 25% of all patients with colorectal cancer, includes serial chest radiography every 6 months and serum carcinoembryonic antigen determinations every 2 to 3 months. Routine surveillance with abdominal or pelvic computed tomography scans has not yet proven to be cost-effective, and liver chemistries are insufficiently sensitive to be of value.

PATIENT SURVEILLANCE FOR CHRONIC INFLAMMATORY BOWEL DISEASE

The incidence of colorectal cancer is substantially increased in patients with long-standing inflammatory bowel disease. Although this increased risk is best defined for chronic ulcerative colitis, patients with long-standing Crohn's disease of the large bowel also have an increased risk. Estimates of cancer incidence in chronic ulcerative colitis vary widely. Estimates from community clinics and population-based studies are probably more accurate than those from referral centers and indicate an annual cancer risk of at least 0.5% per year after the first decade of colitis.

The magnitude of cancer risk in a given patient correlates with the extent and duration of colitis. It is much higher for patients with pancolitis than for patients with disease limited to the left side of the large bowel. Overall, the average relative risk of cancer is increased approximately 14-fold for patients with pancolitis and two- to threefold for left-sided disease. Patients with just proctitis or proctosigmoiditis have a slightly increased risk. Low cancer risk exists during the first 10 years of disease. After 10 years, the risk increases progressively with each decade, and nearly 12 to 15% of patients will develop cancer by 25 years of age unless special surveillance is performed. Although less precisely defined, the risk of colorectal cancer in patients with Crohn's colitis appears to be approximately the same as that of left-sided ulcerative colitis.

Colorectal cancers that arise in patients with inflammatory bowel disease differ in many significant ways from sporadic cancers. Colorectal cancers are more evenly distributed throughout the colon, are three to four times more likely to be multiple at the time of diagnosis, occur at a much younger average age, and nearly 50% are poorly-differentiated histologically. Rather than arising in well-defined benign adenomatous polyps, these cancers commonly arise in neoplastic dysplastic changes in flat mucosa. This dysplasia often precedes or is associated with a cancer, and its identification forms the basis of precancerous colonoscopic surveillance designed to identify which patients will require prophylactic colectomy to prevent fatal cancer.

Dysplasia is histologically classified as being low- or high-grade or indefinite. Outcome studies indicate that up to 42% of patients found to have confirmed high-grade dysplasia already have cancer or will develop it within a short time. Low-grade dysplasia is also highly predictive of cancer, and 19% of patients with low-grade dysplasia have or will develop cancer. The risk of cancer approaches 40% when dysplasia is associated with a raised lesion (dysplasia in a lesion or mass [DALM]). Approximately 18% of patients develop high-grade dysplasia or eventual cancer even when colonoscopic biopsies show indefinite dysplasia. Conversely, the finding of no dysplasia is strongly predictive of a good immediate outcome, and 5% of patients have cancer at the time or develop it shortly after surveillance.

Current guidelines recommend colonoscopic surveillance be offered to patients 7 to 10 years after onset of pancolitis or 12 to 15 years after onset of left-sided ulcerative colitis (Table 5.3). Biopsies should be taken approximately every 10 cm throughout the colon, and any strictured, raised, or velvety-appearing area should be carefully biopsied. Initially, colonoscopy should be repeated every 2 to 3 years because cancer risk is still low. After 20 years of disease, however, the risk of cancer rises to a level that requires patient surveillance every year. Biopsy specimens should be interpreted by a pathologist with experience in this area, and dysplasia should usually be confirmed by a second experienced pathologist before colectomy is recommended.

Because of practical and ethical considerations, there has not been, and probably never will be, a well-designed prospective randomized trial to determine the value of cancer surveillance in patients with chronic ulcerative colitis. Outcome studies, however, show that cancers occurring in patients participating in surveillance programs are much more likely to be detected at an earlier, more favorable stage and patients in whom cancer was detected and who undergo surgical resection have a better 5-year survival rate.

Current guidelines recommend surveillance be continued at 1- to 3-year intervals depending on the duration of disease if

Table 5.3

**ENDOSCOPIC SURVEILLANCE OF PATIENTS WITH
CHRONIC ULCERATIVE COLITIS**

1. Begin surveillance 7 to 10 years after onset of pancolitis and 12 to 15 years after onset of left-sided colitis.
2. Perform colonoscopy with mucosal biopsies every 10 cm and biopsy raised or mass lesions.
3. If no dysplasia is found, repeat procedure every 2 to 3 years and repeat annually after 20 years of disease management.
4. Repeat surveillance in 6 to 12 months if indefinite dysplasia is found.
5. Recommend colectomy for patients with confirmed high-grade dysplasia or dysplasia in a lesion or mass.
6. Strongly consider colectomy for patients with confirmed low-grade dysplasia.

no dysplasia is found at colonoscopy. Yearly surveillance is usually indicated after 20 years. If indefinite dysplasia is reported
by the pathologist, this reading should be confirmed by a second experienced pathologist and then surveillance should be
repeated in 6 to 12 months. The finding of confirmed high-
grade dysplasia or of dysplasia associated with a lesion or mass
is an indication for colectomy. Although more controversial,
most guidelines also currently recommend that colectomy be
strongly considered when confirmed low-grade dysplasia is
found because a substantial percentage of these patients have
or will develop cancer.

Surveillance should only be performed in patients who are
willing and able to undergo a colectomy upon being diagnosed
with dysplasia. The advantages and limitations of surveillance
should be discussed in advance with each patient. It should be
emphasized that surveillance is not completely protective since
5 to 8% of cancers occur in patients in whom no dysplasia has
been found. Even multiple biopsies are capable of sampling
only a minute percentage of the total colonic mucosa, so dysplasia may be present at the time of surveillance examination
but be missed by chance. Some interobserver error exists even
between experienced pathologists. There are no prospective,
randomized studies to guide our practice in this area, and little
reliable information exists about the cost or cost-effectiveness
of this approach.

Each case should be carefully individualized. Very young
patients facing a lifetime of cancer risk, especially if they have
bothersome symptomatic disease, may prefer to undergo a prophylactic colectomy rather than face the uncertainties and
trouble of long-term surveillance. On the other hand, there
may be no need to ever consider surveillance when colitis
begins in older patients because the risk of cancer does not become appreciable until 10 to 15 years later. Since most patients

eventually become relatively asymptomatic from their colitis and because most patients will never develop cancers, the majority of patients with long-term ulcerative colitis choose to have surveillance performed rather than undergo immediate prophylactic colectomy or face the risk of possible cancer later in life with no attempted surveillance protection.

The risk of cancer in patients with Crohn's colitis appears to be also related to the extent and duration of disease. However, a larger percentage of patients with extensive Crohn's disease undergo early surgical colonic resection for symptoms or complications of their disease and therefore will not ever be candidates for colonoscopic surveillance. Less is known about the relation between cancer risk and identifiable precancerous dysplasia in Crohn's disease, and no specific guidelines are available to guide practice. Most experts are beginning to recommend periodic colonoscopic surveillance in patients with extensive Crohn's colitis after 10 years of disease management. Special attention should be directed at new symptoms or the development of a colonic stricture that may be the result of a colorectal cancer arising in patients with Crohn's disease of long duration.

SUMMARY

Colonoscopic surveillance for patients with an above-average risk for adenomatous polyps and colorectal cancer is recommended by current evidence-based practice guidelines. High-risk groups include patients with a personal or family history of colorectal neoplasia and patients with long-standing chronic inflammatory bowel disease involving the large bowel. Surveillance recommendations are based on stratification of each individual's estimated cancer risk, which is derived from a careful analysis of clinical variables that have been identified in recent scientific studies.

SUGGESTED READINGS

Bond JH, the Practice Parameters Committee of the American College of Gastroenterology. Diagnosis, treatment, and surveillance for patients with nonfamilial colorectal polyps. Ann Intern Med 1993;119:836–843. (This guideline prepared by the American College of Gastroenterology and endorsed by other medical gastrointestinal societies outlines evidence-based recommendations for the diagnosis, management, and follow-up surveillance of patients with colorectal adenomatous polyps.)

Buie WD, Rothenberger DA. Surveillance after curative resection of colorectal cancer: Individualizing follow-up. Gastrointest Endosc Clin N Am 1993;3:691–713. (This comprehensive review of data supports recommendations for follow-up surveillance of patients who have had curative surgical resection of colorectal cancers.)

Burt RW, Petersen GM. Familial colorectal cancer: Diagnosis and management. In: Young G, Rozen P, Levin B, eds. Prevention and early detection of colorectal cancer. Philadelphia: W.B. Saunders, 1996:171–194. (This excellent review of the genetics of familial colorectal cancer contains recommendations for surveillance of patients with FAP, nonpolyposis colorectal cancer syndrome, and familial risk for sporadic cancers.)

Lennard-Jones JE. Prevention of cancer mortality in inflammatory bowel disease. In: Prevention and early detection of colorectal cancer. Young GP, Rozen P, Levin B, eds. London: W.B. Saunders, 1996:217–238. (This comprehensive review of data demonstrates the risk of colorectal cancer in patients with chronic ulcerative colitis or Crohn's disease and supports current recommendations for colonoscopic surveillance.)

Winawer SJ, Fletcher RH, Miller L, et al. Colorectal cancer screening: Clinical guidelines and rationale. Gastroenterology 1997;112:594–642. (This is a comprehensive evidence-based practice guideline developed by a multidisciplinary panel of experts under the sponsorship of the Federal Agency for Health Care Policy and Research and a consortium of five medical and surgical gastrointestinal professional societies. It provides recommendations for screening of the average-risk population for colorectal cancer and surveillance of high-risk groups.)

Winawer SJ, Zauber AG, Gerdes H, et al. Risk of colorectal cancer in the families of patients with adenomatous polyps. N Engl J Med 1996;334:82–87. (This data from the National Polyp Study demonstrates an increased risk of colorectal cancer in siblings of selected patients with adenomatous polyps. Recommendations for surveillance of affected patients is provided based on these findings.)

Winawer SJ, Zauber AG, O'Brien MJ, et al. Randomized comparison of surveillance intervals after colonoscopic removal of newly diagnosed adenomatous polyps. N Engl J Med 1993; 328:901–906. (This multicenter controlled trial was designed to determine effective follow-up surveillance of patients who had resection of colorectal adenomatous polyps.)

Chapter 6

EVOLVING THERAPIES FOR COLON CANCER

Lee S. Rosen, MD

INTRODUCTION

In 1996, more than 135,000 new cases of colorectal cancer were diagnosed in the United States and more than 50,000 people died of the disease. The disease is a large public health problem and accounts for nearly 10% of all cancer diagnoses and nearly 10% of all cancer deaths. Early detection substantially impacts survival rates of patients with colorectal cancer, and discussion of colorectal cancer should emphasize proper and routine screening of all patients after assessing relative risk of contracting the disease. This chapter focuses on current understanding of the treatment of patients with colorectal cancer and includes discussions on the benefits of adjuvant therapy in patients with early-stage cancer and summaries of most recent chemotherapy trial results. Where 5-fluorouracil (5FU) or some derivative thereof was once the only treatment for advanced disease. there are newer compounds that show promising activity in resistant and even untreated metastatic disease. In addition, other interventions besides systemic chemotherapy (e.g., monoclonal antibodies, hepatic arterial infusion (HAI), and surgical resection of liver metastases) are reviewed.

ADJUVANT THERAPY

Failure following primary surgical resection of colorectal cancers has warranted therapy improvements. Although patients with colon cancer are more likely to have distant recurrence (mainly located in the liver and lungs), rectal cancers have higher local recurrence rates. Problems obtaining adequate surgical margins in rectal cancer and the lack of a serosal layer in the distal gastrointestinal tract are two reasons for the increased rates of local failures in patients with rectal cancer. Although clinical trials exploring the advantages of adjuvant therapy for colorectal cancer date back to the 1950s, it was not until recently that a therapy showed improved disease-free and overall survival rates. Early studies with single agents like thiotepa, floxuridine (FUDR), and 5FU (administered in inadequate intravenous doses, intraluminally, or orally) failed to demonstrate any clinical benefit. Nearly 3500 patients over an approximate 20-year period were enrolled in these studies. Embedded in these data, however, were trial design limitations, which included the combination of patients with colon and rectal cancer (of several different stages) and failure to use uniform staging or surgical procedures.

COMBINATION CHEMOTHERAPY

Improvements in drug delivery also aided the next generation of studies. These studies were mainly combination chemotherapy trials and commonly included 5FU with methyl-lomustine treatments. A statistically significant improvement in disease-free and overall survival rates was seen in the National Surgical Adjuvant Breast and Bowel Projects (NSABP) C01 study, which was first reported in 1988. In this study, 5FU, vincristine, and methotrexate treatment was superior to observation or immunotherapy (Bacillus Calmette-Guérin [BCG]). Unfortunately, the use of methotrexate was associated with an increased incidence of myelodysplasia or leukemia, and its routine use was abandoned. Other trials failed to confirm these results, and slightly different drug treatment schedules and entry criteria may have played a role in the trials' unsuccessful results.

PORTAL VEIN CHEMOTHERAPY

Researchers studied the administration of 5FU treatment directly into the portal vein because of the high rate of relapses isolated to the liver. Several randomized trials compared postoperative portal vein infusions of 5FU (with or without heparin) to surgery alone and failed to demonstrate statistically significant advantages in hepatic recurrence or overall survival rates. The NSABP C02 study, which was conducted in 1990 and updated 4 years later, enrolled 1158 patients who were randomly assigned to surgery or 7 days of postoperative portal vein infusions of 5FU/heparin treatment. The chemotherapy patients had an improved disease-free survival rate (68% versus 60%, $P = .01$) and overall survival rate (76% versus 71%, $P = .03$). There was no difference in hepatic recurrence rates, leading the authors of the study to conclude advantages seen in the treatment group were the result of the systemic effects of 5FU treatment. All of the adjuvant portal vein therapy trials can be criticized because of their broad inclusion criteria of enrolling patients with Dukes' A, B, and C cancers together. Considering the data available today, it seems the duration of adjuvant therapy was suboptimal.

LEVAMISOLE

The antihelminthic agent levamisole had been studied in patients with advanced colorectal cancer and did not show any advantage over 5FU treatment alone. Verhaegen first used levamisole alone as adjuvant therapy for patients with advanced colorectal cancer because of the immunomodulatory properties that were demonstrated in the laboratory. In a small non-randomized study of patients with Dukes' A, B, and C cancer, a higher overall survival rate in the levamisole-treated group was demonstrated compared to the group treated with surgery alone. Other subsequent and prospective, randomized, placebo-controlled studies failed to show an advantage to single-agent levamisole over observation alone. Moertel et al's pivotal study, which was reported in 1990 and updated in 1995, demonstrated a 40% improvement in disease-free survival rates ($P < .0001$) and a 33% improvement in overall survival rates ($P = .0007$) for patients with Dukes' C cancer who were treated with 12 months of 5FU/levamisole therapy compared to patients treated with surgery alone. No statistically significant advantage was seen to levamisole treatment alone. The standard of care in patients with Dukes' C cancer quickly became the 12-month regimen of 5FU/levamisole. However, no prospective randomized study has ever shown an advantage of 5FU/levamisole treatment over 5FU alone.

LEUCOVORIN-CONTAINING REGIMENS

The NSABP C03 trial, which was reported in 1993, showed the superiority of a 12-month treatment regimen of 5FU/leucovorin over methotrexate, vincristine, and 5FU (MOF). The International Multicenter Pooled Analysis of Colon Cancer Trials (IMPACT) and another study reported in a 1993 abstract and 1997 article enrolled 317 patients with Dukes' B3 and C tumors. These studies also showed the advantage of a 6-month treatment regimen of 5FU/leucovorin over surgery alone. Treated patients had longer 5-year disease-free survival rates (74% versus 58%, $P < .01$) and higher overall survival rates (74% versus 63%, $P = .02$). All of these results confirm the advantage of some type of 5FU-based therapy in patients who are node-positive (Dukes' C), suggest a similar trend in patients with Dukes' B2 and B3 cancer, and virtually eliminate the need for surgery-alone control groups.

RECENTLY COMPLETED COMPARISON TRIALS

The large trials discussed above opened the door for comparisons between leucovorin- and levamisole-containing regimens and between various schedules and durations of therapy. The NSABP C04 trial compared 5FU/leucovorin treatment, 5FU/levamisole treatment, and 5FU/leucovorin/levamisole treatment and enrolled 2151 patients with Dukes' B and C cancer between 1989 and 1990. Five-year disease-free survival rates were 64%, 64%, and 60% ($P = $ NS), respectively, and 5-year overall survival rates were 74%, 72%, and 69% ($P = $ NS), respectively. The benefits of one particular treatment regimen may emerge with greater maturity of the data and a more detailed subset analysis. The National Cancer Institute of Canada and the North Central Cancer Treatment Group reported a 2 × 2 randomized trial designed to compare 6 months to 12 months of adjuvant chemotherapy and 5FU/levamisole to 5FU/leucovorin/levamisole treatment. These data were presented at the American Society of Clinical Oncology (ASCO) annual meeting in 1996 and showed that 12 months of therapy conferred no advantage over 6 months and a 6-month treatment regimen of 5FU/leucovorin/levamisole was associated with the highest survival rates but was not significantly superior to either regimen when administered for 12 months.

These trials and others can be confusing to the practicing physician. Unfortunately, little uniformity in chemotherapy schedules or drug combinations exist because of the extreme length of time for studies such as these to mature. The Intergroup 0089 study, which was designed in 1988, was a prospective randomized trial that also attempted to clarify the optimal adjuvant therapy regimen for patients with colorectal cancer. The Intergroup 0089 study initially sought to compare surgery alone with a 6-month treatment regimen of 5FU with high dose leucovorin (weekly bolus infusion schedule) or a 6-month treatment regimen of 5FU with low dose leucovorin (bolus infusions 5 days in a row administered every 4 weeks). The group undergoing surgery alone was terminated when Moertel's study was completed in 1989, and groups using the 5FU/levamisole regimen and the 5FU/leucovorin/levamisole combination were added. Preliminary results were presented at the 1996 ASCO meeting and updated a year later. Adding levamisole therapy confers no advantage to the 5FU with low dose leucovorin treatment regimen, and a 6-month treatment regimen of 5FU/leucovorin (high or low dose) is as effective as a 12-month treatment regimen of 5FU/levamisole. The only group remaining to be analyzed compares the 5FU/levamisole treatment regimen to the 5FU/leucovorin/levamisole treatment regimen.

SUMMARY

Possible treatment modalities for patients with Dukes' B2, B3, and C cancer include enrollment in a well-designed clinical trial or treatment with a type of 5FU-based adjuvant therapy (12-month treatment regimen of 5FU/levamisole or a 6-month treatment regimen of 5FU/leucovorin). Ongoing trials and recently completed trials are attempting to define the optimal treatment regimen and schedule and explore the precise perioperative timing of adjuvant therapy. Finally, recent data suggesting an advantage to protracted rather than bolus infusion of 5FU have led to another generation of intergroup studies.

Prognostic variables may also help clarify which patients should receive adjuvant therapy. The Deleted in Colon Cancer (DCC) gene is a deletion in the long arm of chromosome 18 (18q-). Recently, a retrospective immunohistochemical analysis of Dukes' B tumor samples reported patients whose tumors expressed the abnormal gene product had a risk of disease-relapse similar to their counterparts with node-positive disease.

THERAPY FOR ADVANCED DISEASE

The treatment of choice for patients with initially advanced or recurrent colorectal cancer is 5FU-based therapy. Single agent studies dating back to the 1960s have shown response rates ranging from 8 to 85%. Toxicity profiles and perhaps mechanisms of action can be altered by delivering 5FU through bolus infusion or continuous infusion using a portable pump. Leucovorin modulation enhances the effectiveness of 5FU treatment by stabilizing the thymidylate synthase(TS)/FdUMP complex. The octopus study reported by the Southwest Oncology Group in 1995 failed to show improved survival or response rates to any of several 5FU regimens with or without bolus or continuous infusion leucovorin.

Recent research conducted by Lenz et al reported tumor expression of TS in patients with advanced disease can predict clinical response to 5FU-based therapy. Approximately 53% (10/19) of patients with TS levels ≤ 3.5 responded to therapy compared to 0% (0/18) of patients with TS levels above 3.5 ($P < .001$) Lenz et al also suggested a correlation between high TS levels and expression of the mutant p53 tumor suppressor gene. This same study retrospectively looked at immunohistochemically-stained tumor samples of patients receiving adjuvant therapy or therapy for advanced disease in large clinical trials. High qualitative staining scores for TS levels predicted poorer survival rates and poorer response rates to therapy. Furthermore, a subset analysis of patients with high TS levels in the adjuvant trials failed to show improved disease-free or overall survival rates with or without adjuvant therapy.

CAMPTOTHECINS

Irinotecan (CPT11), a topoisomerase I inhibitor, is a semisynthetic derivative of the Camptotheca acuminata tree. The plant alkaloid, camptothecin, was first identified in the 1960s as part of a broad screen of natural products and was found to have significant in vitro anticancer effects. The drug was abandoned, however, because of severe side effects. In the 1980s, researchers discovered camptothecin inhibits topoisomerase I, which is an enzyme that allows relaxation of the double stranded DNA's torsional strain as it unwinds to begin replication. CPT11 and its metabolite, SN38, prevent DNA relegation following single-strand breakage (the cleaveable complex) caused by topoisomerase I. The chemical structure of CPT11 and its rapid in vivo de-esterification to SN38 enhances its efficacy while avoiding many of the systemic side effects of its predecessors.

Several phase I trials provide the rationale for current dosing schedules of CPT11. In the United States, CPT11 treatment is administered weekly for 4 weeks as a 90-minute 125 mg/m^2 infusion and is followed by a 2 week rest. The drug is routinely administered in Europe as 350 mg/m^2 over 30 minutes every 3 weeks. Continuous infusion schedules have been tested, and no data have resulted to support theories of improved efficacy or decreased toxicity. The main side effects of CPT11 include diarrhea (which can be managed effectively by a high dose loperamide regimen developed by Abigerges et al), leukopenia, mild nausea, fatigue, and alopecia. In addition, patients may experience sweating, flushing, abdominal cramping, nausea, and vomiting during or immediately following drug infusion. This cholinergic reaction is thought to be the result of CPT11's inhibition of cholinesterase and is more common with higher doses or more rapid infusions. Administration of 0.25 to 1 mg of atropine alleviates the symptoms almost immediately. CPT11 treatment should be avoided in patients with severe renal or hepatic insufficiency because of inadequate data on the drug metabolism in that patient group.

Rothenberg et al reported the results of a phase II trial on a 90-minute 125 mg/m^2 CPT11 infusion, which was administered weekly for 4 weeks and followed by a 2 week rest, in patients with metastatic colorectal cancer that had progressed within 6 months of one previous 5FU treatment regimen. Of 48 patients entered into the study, one patient completely responded to treatment and nine patients partially responded to treatment (response rate 23%, 95% confidence interval [CI] = 10 to 36%). An additional fifteen patients (31%) had stable disease that lasted more than 4 months (range 4 to 16). The median survival rate of all patients was 10.4 months. The North Central Cancer Treatment group also reported a phase II trial using the identical schedule that consisted of 121 patients, 90 of which had a history of 5FU therapy and 31 of which had no history of chemotherapy. A response rate of 13.3% (95% CI = 7.1 to 22.1%) in pretreated patients and 25.8% (95% CI = 11.9 to 44.6%) in untreated patients compares favorably with Rothenberg's findings. Response duration in both groups was approximately 7.5 months (range 2.8 to 31.7).

The response rates reported in the early phase II trials are similar to those seen with 5FU therapy in untreated patients. Although the rates were low and short survival periods were recorded, the rates in patients with 5FU-refractory disease were improvements over the standard of care and led to rapid Food and Drug Administration (FDA) approval. Van Cutsam et al in Belgium presented data about CPT11's clinical benefit at the 1997 ASCO meeting. The median survival rate was 9.5 months in the 455 patients treated with CPT11, and the survival rate was 14.5 months in responders and 12.5 months in the 42% of patients with stable disease. CPT11 may improve survival rates and quality of life (defined as decreased analgesic consumption) in patients with stable disease rather than only in those with traditionally defined complete and partial responses.

CPT11 therapy represents a major breakthrough in the treatment of patients with colorectal cancer by offering an effective agent besides 5FU. Patients' adequate performance status, ability to manage diarrhea, and sufficient hepatic, renal, and bone marrow reserve is the key to effective drug treatment. Studies are evaluating different drug treatment schedules and the role of CPT11 treatment alone or administered with 5FU in patients with untreated metastatic disease. Other camptothecins, including topotecan and 9-aminocamptothecin, do not appear to be active in the treatment of colorectal cancer in the schedules.

OXALIPLATIN

Oxaliplatin is a new platinum analog that also has in vitro activity against colorectal cancer cell lines. As a single agent, response rates of 10% were reported in patients with metastatic disease refractory to 5FU treatment. Phase II trials suggest the response rate of oxaliplatin as a single agent treatment in patients with untreated metastatic colorectal cancer may be as high as 20%. Added to 5FU, however, oxaliplatin may have superior efficacy rates. Levi et al reported the oxaliplatin with 5FU/leucovorin combination has response rates of 28% in previously treated patients and up to 53% (95% CI = 38 to 68%) in chemotherapy-naive patients. In the former group, the 28% salvage rate was seen when oxaliplatin was added to the same 5FU-containing regimen on which the patients had just progressed. The reason for the responses are unclear but suggest some drug interaction whereby oxaliplatin reverses 5FU resistance in patients.

Most of the research on oxaliplatin, which is commercially available in Europe but investigational in the United States, comes from studies with chronomodulation conducted by Levi et al. Levi reported the results of a randomized trial comparing constant-rate continuous infusion 5FU/leucovorin/oxaliplatin treatment with infusional 5FU/leucovorin/oxaliplatin doses adjusted for the body's circadian rhythms (maximum delivery of 5FU at 4AM and maximum delivery of oxaliplatin at 4PM). The chronomodulated group had improved response rates (53% [95% CI = 38 to 68%] versus 32% [95% CI = 18 to 46%]) and improved survival rates (9 months [95% CI = 0.8 to 23.2%]) versus 14.9 months [95% CI = 12.1 to 17.8]). Chronomodulation also reduces toxicity, which allows for overall higher doses of chemotherapy. Levi et al continue to experiment with different chronomodulation schedules and chemotherapy doses. In the United States, oxaliplatin is being evaluated in a multi-center trial of patients with untreated metastatic disease and patients within 2 months of disease progression on a 5FU-based regimen (oxaliplatin added to the same 5FU-containing regimen the patient was treated with but without chronomodulation). Side effects of oxaliplatin include nausea, vomiting, diarrhea, and peripheral neuropathies.

LY231514

LY231514, a multi-targeted folate antagonist, blocks TS, dihydrofolate reductase (DHFR), and glycinamide ribonucleotide formyltransferase (GARFT). These enzymes are involved in purine biosynthesis. The drug's main side effects appear to be myelosuppression, mucositis, diarrhea, and rash. Phase I trials have been performed to determine maximum tolerated dosing on different schedules, and early phase II results have been reported in abstracts. In May 1997, Cripps et al described a response rate of 23% (95% CI = 10 to 42%) in patients with metastatic colorectal cancer who were intravenously treated with 500 to 600 mg/m^2 of LY231514 every 3 weeks. Larger confirmatory trials are currently underway.

MONOCLONAL ANTIBODIES

In 1994, Riethmüller et al reported the results of a randomized trial in patients with Dukes' C colorectal cancer that compared observation alone to administration of monoclonal antibody 17–1A. The 189 patients were randomized postoperatively, and the 90 patients in the treatment group received 500 mg of antibody treatment 2 weeks after surgery and 4 monthly infusions of 100 mg thereafter. No patient in either group received adjuvant chemotherapy or radiotherapy. After a median follow-up of 5 years, patients who received antibody 17–1A had a 30% decrease in the overall death rate ($P = .05$) and a 27% decrease in the recurrence rate ($P = .05$). Side effects were mild and consisted of fatigue, nausea, and diarrhea. The data were updated in May 1996 and confirmed the results at 7 years. Trials are underway, mainly in Europe, to evaluate the difference between traditional 5FU-based adjuvant therapy and 5FU-based therapy combined with the antibody.

Other antibodies are also currently being studied. A phase I trial of a superantigen-based immunotherapy, PNU-214565, was recently completed and showed a single dose of this agent was tolerated safely. PNU-214565 hopes to induce an antitumor immune response independent of major histocompatibility complex (MHC) class II expression patterns. An anti-carcinoembryonic antigen (CEA) monoclonal antibody is also being evaluated in clinical trials at multiple sites in the United States.

HEPATIC ARTERIAL CHEMOTHERAPY

Up to 50,000 patients will be diagnosed with liver metastases from colorectal cancer each year in the United States. At autopsy, slightly more than 33% of patients will have their only metastases in the liver. The fluoropyrimidines can be administered through HAI. FUDR is metabolized in the liver with a high hepatic extraction rate and little systemic absorption; in this way, higher doses of the agent can be safely administered to patients. Although initial phase II studies reported response rates of 30 to 78%, there have been randomized trials that confirm higher response rates to HAI than to intravenous 5FU but no significant survival advantage. Crossover was allowed in most trials, which made the data even harder to interpret. Rougier et al reported in 1992 the results of a prospective randomized trial comparing HAI FUDR treatment, systemic 5FU treatment, and observation alone in patients with metastatic disease confined to the liver. No crossover was permitted, but patients in the systemic chemotherapy group were not treated uniformly. The HAI group had a response rate of 43% versus

9% in the group treated with 5FU alone. A statistically significant increase in survival rates was also seen in the HAI group.

Side effects of HAI therapy are problems related to catheter placement, elevations in liver enzyme levels, biliary sclerosis, infection, and thromboses. Newer infusion pumps and chemotherapy combinations have been tested to ameliorate these toxicities. Kemeny et al added dexamethasone to FUDR treatment and then dexamethasone and leucovorin to FUDR treatment. Kemeny et al claimed a 78% response rate and a 3% incidence of biliary sclerosis in the approximately 35 patients who were enrolled in a phase II trial of the latter combination. In a phase II trial by Patt et al of HAI treatment with 5FU (not FUDR) and α-interferon, researchers attempted to take advantage of the biologic modifier's in vitro synergism with 5FU and its antiangiogenic properties. Although this regimen was tolerated and no hepatobiliary toxicity was seen in the 48 patients enrolled in the study, the response rate was 33.3% (95% CI = 20 to 49%) and the median response duration was 7 months. All patients enrolled in the study were pretreated patients. The future of this regimen remains doubtful because larger scale systemic regimens show no advantage to the addition of interferon to 5FU-based therapy. Future trials to optimize HAI chemotherapy regimens or combine them with other systemic therapies are planned.

RESECTION OF LIVER METASTASES

Surgical excision of the liver lesion(s) in the appropriate patient can improve survival rates because metastatic disease is confined to the liver in many patients. Fong et al reviewed 456 patients treated from 1985 to 1991in a single-institution who had adequate hepatic reserve following surgery, no signs of disease outside the liver, and no major comorbid medical conditions. The patient group's perioperative mortality rate was 3%, morbidity rate, 31% (mainly infections), 5-year disease-free survival rate, 19%, and 5-year overall survival rate, 38%. Many other series describe similar survival rates. Hughes et al published results of 607 patients who had a 5-year survival rate of 33%. At least ten other series, with study groups ranging from 20 to 250 patients, describe 5-year survival rates ranging from 22 to 45%. These numbers compare quite favorably to historic control groups treated with chemotherapy alone. No prospective randomized trials have been performed, and prospective randomized trials will probably never be done.

Fong et al and other studies attempt to define clinical features that would predict adverse outcomes in patients. Some features are obvious and include number of metastases, size of the resected metastases, short disease-free survival rates before surgery, and elevated preoperative CEA levels. However, none of the possible poor prognostic factors precluded long-term survival in all patients of a particular subgroup. The only definitive contraindication to hepatic resection was extra-hepatic disease. Fong et al advocate considering all patients with disease confined to the liver for surgical resection and suggest future clinical trials be performed to evaluate the role of postresection adjuvant systemic or regional chemotherapy.

CONCLUSION

For several years now, researchers have failed to improve upon 5FU-based therapy as treatment of patients with advanced disease or to clarify the duration and schedule of therapy in earlier-stage patients. Overall survival rates of less than 2 years in patients with metastatic disease are unacceptable. Hopefully, the new agents, new types of therapy, and improved combined modality therapies will lead to greater survival rates, improved quality of life, and even cures.

SUGGESTED READINGS

Bertheault-Cvitkovic F, Jami A, Ithzaki M, et al. Biweekly intensified ambulatory chronomodulated chemotherapy with oxaliplatin, fluorouracil, and leucovorin in patients with metastatic colorectal cancer. J Clin Oncol 1996;14:2950–2958. (This recent report from the Levi et al group discusses chronomodulation and use of oxaliplatin.)

Fong Y, Cohen AM, Fortner JG, et al. Liver resection for colorectal metastases. J Clin Oncol 1997;15:938–946. (This article consists of a single institution review of 456 consecutive resections in patients with liver metastases from colorectal cancer and contains a discussion of the therapy modality genes as the basis for this report.)

Leichman L, Lenz HJ, Leichman CG, et al. Quantitation of intratumoral thymidylate synthase expression predicts for resistance to protracted infusion of 5-fluorouracil and weekly leucovorin in disseminated colorectal cancers: preliminary report from an ongoing trial. Euro J Cancer 1995;31A:1306–1310. (This preliminary report of the group's work suggests a correlation between TS levels in colorectal tumors and patients' response to therapy. Many updates have been recorded in abstracts since publication of this article.)

O'Connell M, Mailliard J, Kahn M, et al. Controlled trial of fluorouracil and low dose leucovorin given for 6 months as postoperative adjuvant therapy for colon cancer. J Clin Oncol 1997;15:246–250. (Results show success with 6 months of a 5FU/leucovorin adjuvant regimen is different than the other regimen of 12 months of 5FU/levamisole.)

Riethmuller G, Schneider-Gadicke E, Schlimok G, et al. Randomized trial of monoclonal antibody for adjuvant therapy of resected Dukes' C colorectal carcinoma. Lancet 1994;343:1177–1183. (This is the first prospective, randomized clinical trial showing improved disease-free and overall survival rates to antibody 17–1A in patients with Dukes' C cancer.)

Rothenberg ML, Eckardt JR, Kuhn JG, et al. Phase II trial of Irinotecan in patients with progressive or rapidly recurrent colorectal cancer. J Clin Oncol 1996;14:1128–1135. (A pivotal phase II trial that demonstrates the efficacy of CPT11 in metastatic colorectal cancer refractory to 5FU.)

Shibata D, Reale MA, Lavin P, et al. The DCC protein and prognosis in colorectal cancer. N Engl J Med 1996;335:1727–1732. (This article reviews immunohistochemical analysis of 132 colorectal cancer tissues for expression of the DCC gene. Patients with aberrant expression had a worse prognosis than those who did not.)

Index